HYDROSOL THERAPY

of related interest

Essential Oils 3rd Edition (forthcoming)
Jennifer Peace Rhind
ISBN 978 1 84819 385 7
eISBN 978 0 85701 343 9

Seven Scents
Healing and the Aromatic Imagination
Dorothy P. Abram
Illustrated by Laura Mernoff
ISBN 978 1 84819 349 9
eISBN 978 0 85701 307 1

Listening to Scent
An Olfactory Journey with Aromatic Plants and Their Extracts
Jennifer Peace Rhind
ISBN 978 1 84819 125 9
eISBN 978 0 85701 171 8

Aromatica
A Clinical Guide to Essential Oil Therapeutics
Volume 1: Principles and Profiles
Peter Holmes
ISBN 978 1 84819 303 1
eISBN 978 0 85701 257 9

Aromatherapeutic Blending
Essential Oils in Synergy
Jennifer Peace Rhind
ISBN 978 1 84819 303 1
eISBN 978 0 85701 257 9

HYDROSOL THERAPY

A Handbook for Aromatherapists and Other Practitioners

— *Lydia Bosson* —

Translated by Jonathan Hinde

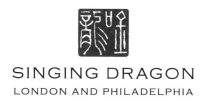

SINGING DRAGON

LONDON AND PHILADELPHIA

First published in 2019
by Jessica Kingsley Publishers
73 Collier Street
London N1 9BE, UK
and
400 Market Street, Suite 400
Philadelphia, PA 19106, USA

www.jkp.com

Edition originale en langue française
Hydrolathérapie – Guérir avec les eaux subtiles des plantes.
© Editions Amyris SPRL
22 rue Lannoy – 1050 Bruxelles
Site internet: www.editionsamyris.com
Conception de la collection: Bénédicte Jeunehomme
Dépôt légal: D2015/7706/116

Library of Congress Cataloging in Publication Data
A CIP catalog record for this book is available from the Library of Congress

British Library Cataloguing in Publication Data
A CIP catalogue record for this book is available from the British Library

ISBN 978 1 84819 423 6
eISBN 978 0 85701 384 2

Printed and bound in the Great Britain

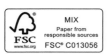

This book is dedicated to my British family, especially to my father, Norman Alan Clewlow and my brother Philip Clewlow, who unfortunately, I've never met. Wherever you are in this universe, know that you are always in my heart.

CONTENTS

Acknowledgements

Writing a book about remedies or therapies takes a team, and it is collective endeavour based on the experience and knowledge we learned together. It is also an evolving project, requiring the transmission of learned knowledge and sometimes allowing inspiration to guide us down new paths. At certain times, we learned new things and this pushed us to explore more deeply a new subject. I was extremely lucky to be surrounded by extraordinary people.

I am deeply thankful to the sessional professors at Usha Veda holistic college, recognised therapists and experts in the field of aroma-phytotherapy and hydrosol therapy. Their passion for transmission of knowledge is a great gift for those who participate in their courses. The experiences of the students are extremely precious. The students' experience is invaluable, as the teaching makes everything so clear and understandable. Above all, a big thank you to my teammates Catherine, Jacqueline and Patricia, who have shared my passion for plants and natural therapies over the past 20 years. Your devotion and loyalty have contributed greatly to my personal growth.

Thank you to our course participants, who have worked with us in this adventure with hydrosols, essential oils and Ayurveda. You are my source of inspiration, and your commitment gives me wings!

Thank you to my dearest friend from Taiwan, Yo June, and the team from Canjune. You have given me the opportunity to discover exceptional hydrosols, such as shiso and champaca. Being able to teach throughout Asia via your training centre fills me with great joy and gratitude. Your trust and enthusiasm motivates me to go beyond my limits.

If today I have the privilege to share my knowledge and passion around the world, it is above all thanks to the love and faith that my family has in this unique story about plants. My life is full of gratitude for my family, my staff and the people who have shared this adventure of spreading the knowledge of plants.

Big thanks to Martine, my sister-in-law, for her joy and organisational skills. To Alexandre, my son and first test subject, for his creativity and important communications advice. And, of course, huge thanks to Philippe, my husband since the start of this adventure, for his continuous support, perseverance and perspicacity.

There are no words to say how much I appreciate the help of Jonathan Hinde. His precious corrections gave a British 'polish' to my book. The endeavour of Jonathan and his wife Mary allowed me to create the connection with the country of my birth, the United Kingdom. Due to their efforts, I have been able to conduct courses in London and reconnect with my roots. Big thanks to Jonathan, Mary and all my British friends for their commitment and, last but not least, their British humour.

A special thanks to the producers from around the world who supply us with these marvellous and precious hydrosols and essential oils. I would like to thank you in advance for all the new marvels that you'll be releasing over the coming years.

Finally, thank you to nature, which supplies us with this huge variety of plants that support and heal us and help us grow.

Discover our activities and our training programs on our site: www.ushaveda.com.

PREFACE

Drop by drop, water sculpts the rock.

— *Theocritus* —

I have been teaching aromatherapy since 1993 and I've always had a strong attraction to hydrosols, which I have used right from the start.

Despite this, when, in 2004, my editors asked me to write a book on the topic I felt like a pioneer in virgin territory, even though my close work with holistic therapists and a good deal of personal experience with hydrosols meant that I already had a good base to work from.

With the passage of time there has been an increase of general interest in these magical waters, which, combined with their availability in greater variety, has resulted in hydrosols becoming an integral part of aromatherapy and herbal medicine.

At the same time, my daily work with hydrosols has allowed me to learn new secrets and has motivated me to further deepen my work. So now seems the perfect time to bring everything to fruition and put it into the form of a book.

Hydrosols and essential oils contain all the 'energy information' from plants. We can think of distillation as a transformative process that frees the most subtle elements from the plant: its essence, its soul. From this perspective, it is perhaps no surprise to see the amazing changes that hydrosols can bring about, both at the psycho-emotional and physical levels.

Putting your trust in plants and their magical waters is something that raises awareness and supports the evolution and healing of the body and mind. Hydrosols are important health remedies because they can easily be integrated into daily life, have few contraindications, and frequently produce huge therapeutic benefit.

Furthermore, hydrosol therapy can be integrated into Chinese medicine, Ayurveda, naturopathy and so on, and it combines perfectly with other herbal medicine approaches. Hydrosols are extremely powerful and often trigger radical changes at both psycho-emotional and physical levels. Given the minute concentration of aromatic molecules, this effect is perhaps difficult to explain, but it seems that they are significant messengers of the plants.

My hope is that this book will be a celebration of the therapeutic qualities and subtle energy of hydrosols, so that plants can fulfil our lives and trigger a fundamental process of healing.

Be humble in the face of the universe

Human behaviour flows from three main sources: desire, emotion, and knowledge.

— *Plato* —

As a child, I particularly loved my grandmother. She was a Greek woman with a strong temperament, a professor of maths and orthodox theology, with a strong vein of faith. She fought for a world without war and practised daily rituals, prayers and meditation. For a while she was even an Orthodox nun. One day when I was about 10 years old, I was walking with her along the beach and I asked her what she did to feel the presence of God. 'You cannot understand God intellectually with your mind. You can only feel God with your heart,' she answered. Then she told me that one of mankind's greatest sins is that he wants at all costs to explain spirituality through the intellect. 'Mankind puts everything that has to do with the intellect and Cartesianism on a pedestal and denigrates everything else. His understanding of things has become egocentric and limited,' she told me.

Our discussion stopped at this stage, but a few years later she told me that there are 7 levels of consciousness in the universe. As there are 7 days of the week, 7 musical notes, 7 colours in the rainbow, 7 deadly sins, 7 chakras, a 7-branched candlestick in the Hebrew tradition and, in another register, 7 wonders of the world, there are also 7 worlds: minerals, plants, animals, humans, angels, archangels and finally God. 'Man is at the centre of these worlds. He is like the 4th chakra. If he knows how to communicate with minerals then he also knows how to communicate with God, and vice versa. But he cannot communicate with a mineral or with God intellectually. He can perceive with the heart, because the heart is the centre of everything that exists in the universe.' On the basis of my understanding today, I say that the heart is the 4th chakra: it connects the 3 lower and 3 upper chakras.

In seeking to understand things with simply the intellect, man limits himself, and his field of vision is reduced. In reality, the size and understanding of the universe is so much bigger than the intellect can appreciate. Now God is in everything, as many spiritual traditions are teaching us. You can understand the stone that you see with your head, you can determine the chemical components that give it mass, but you can also simply 'feel' the rock. And it is only there that you can understand its divine dimension.

My uncle, a surgeon by profession, inherited my grandmother's wisdom. He used to say, 'The Greeks invented the light but they have kept the candle.' I would apply this saying to all humanity. In today's world, it often happens that what is not explained scientifically in accordance with the intellectual understanding of that moment in time is somehow forbidden to exist in the collective consciousness. With this single mechanism, man has created his first prison. It is the same with plants. It is possible to understand one aspect of a plant such as its aroma, its physical virtues or its biochemical composition, but we can understand the plant or its essential oil or hydrosol in its entirety and in all its aspects only if we experience all levels of consciousness. I have made this the precept of life, my mission on earth.

After nourishing my intellect from a scientific perspective, which included understanding the biochemistry of plants, I wanted to feel and experience the essential oils and the hydrosols both with my head and with my heart. I started to read and study everything that came my way concerning different aspects of plants. If a plant is mentioned in history, mythology, legend or even in a grandmother's recipe, I try to understand the symbolism behind that and try to sense it.

I have taken courses on aromatherapy all around the world, but my real breakthroughs have always been the result of the practices of meditation and prayer, together with spiritual workshops focused on intuitive abilities and holistic vision. At the same time, the practical experience of all the therapists who have trusted me for many years has helped me grow and integrate more and more knowledge. I want to thank them for allowing me to publish some of their experiences.

In speaking of gratitude, I can only thank heaven for having spoiled me so much. I am privileged to be surrounded by a lovely and supportive family, to have a team of amazing teachers in my school, with loyal staff, and to have had the chance to meet some outstanding masters in the field of self-development, natural medicine and Ayurveda. And last, but not least, to have the devotion and enthusiasm of my students to contribute to a better world. All these give me the chance to continue with passion and love to promote this message of the soul of plants.

Nature will give you back a hundredfold if you support and defend her beauty. If you trust nature and ultimately life, you break the limitations of the mind, giving up the bad habits of a self-centred intellect. It is important to learn humility and to accept that there may be unknown dimensions.

I am an apprentice of this process of life, and the message of the soul of plants. The herbal world has so much to give us. But even if this way of learning is an endless path, it is pure passion, joy and love. I hope that this knowledge can help you to plant some more seeds for a better world.

Lydia Bosson

Preface to the English Edition

Different Ways to Approach Aroma- and Hydrosol Therapy

As always in the medical approaches, the methods can vary according to the cultures and according to the therapists that they exercise it. There are analogies and sometimes contradictions. The practice of Ayurveda in northern India does not match the way this medicine is applied in the South of the country. There are common bases and different points of view and it's the same with all the other therapeutic approaches around the world. Today, in aromatherapy we speak of a French model and an Anglo-Saxon model, sometimes even of a German model.

From my point of view each approach contains interesting aspects and if we can learn from each other how to combine different methods, then we become more efficient and relevant. It is obvious that this requires in-depth and complex knowledge that neither a book nor a small workshop can replace.

Today when you go to a pharmacy in Geneva or Lausanne and you ask for an allopathic anti-inflammatory drug, the pharmacist might instead recommend to you eucalyptus citriodora to apply without dilution and also to use internally. What can be very common in some parts of the world can be considered as "dangerous" or "unethical" in others.

Different approaches are not better or worse, they lead to different methods of application. Personally, I love to merge different ways and on the other hand I like to observe as Ayurveda taught me. While the approach of aromatherapy in the English-speaking part of this world is often based on external application with massage and skincare, the French school is oriented more towards a phyto-allopathic approach.

The English model has spread all over the world. When I gave my first workshop in Asia I was surprised how much I shocked my students when I was simply saying that you can ingest one drop of cardamom essential oil after a heavy meal or you can rub your armpits with some drops of black spruce when you feel tired. With a deeper understanding of the knowledge and of the biochemical structure of the essential oils, the participants achieve more confidence and could merge with wisdom the different methods.

Today the offer on the world market of essential oils is huge and the numbers of available hydrosols is also increasing drastically. Of course, essential oils are very powerful remedies and as all very effective medicines they can have side-effects. However, every single essential oil has his own biochemical structure, which will determine on the one hand the therapeutic indications and on the other hand if there are precautions to take or side-effects. While certain molecules such as linalool (which is a main component in essential oils like true lavender, rosewood, ho wood etc.) is very well tolerated and has more or less no side effects, it is true that there are also essential oils which can be dangerous especially the ones containing ketones (sage, hyssop, etc.) or phenols (clove, thyme thymol, savory, etc.). It goes without saying that these products can be only used with a professional advice.

From my point of view, it is absurd to discuss whether one can use pure essential oils on the skin or take them internally. The question is rather do we have the knowledge to practice aroma- and hydrosol-therapy safely. Having the necessary education doesn't mean you have to take them absolutely in this or that way, but it does provide the necessary basis to be effective and safe at the same time. It is wonderful to get an aromatherapy massage and it is true, in this case a low concentration of essential oils is just perfect, enjoying a bath with a few drops rosemary borneon and some sea salt is a real detox and boosts our energy. However, massaging the foot soles with a blend of pure essential oils can be very effective and can avoid the use of antibiotics in case of flu, ingesting essential oils like Brazilian pepper (*Schinus terebenthifolius*) with some honey can bring a lot of relief in cases of cough and bronchitis and hence avoid drugs containing codeine. There are numerous examples like this. As the essential oils are powerful, high dilution can still be very effective but in my experience I have often seen that they are not effective in acute cases and then because there is so much fear and a lack of knowledge, people instead take antibiotics, codeine, cortisone etc. which can often be much more harmful for our health.

When I talk with my students about their concerns about how to use essential oils and hydrosols in the best way they often tell me of their difficulty in choosing the right way, being safe and effective at the same time, the right posology, the right rhythm and application. The truth is that you will not be a good therapist just from education; you will become a good one when you achieve experience. To reach this goal, it is important to be aware of different points of view, having the possibility to look to a situation from different angles, having the will to grow and to evolve continuously. I am happy today that I can fulfil the wish of my students to have my first book translated in English. I hope that this book can contribute to some more tools for the therapists, practitioners and all the people who are passionate about these wonderful gifts from Mother Nature.

INTRODUCTION

Only water is eternal.

— Yun Son-Do —

Hydrosols are liquid products coming from the water distillation or steam distillation of plants. They are created at the same time as essential oils, and are also known as hydrosols or floral waters, especially when the distillation comes from flowers, for example with rose or orange blossom. Hydrosol therapy is part of herbal medicine and aromatherapy. The active ingredients in hydrosols are not identical to those of essential oils, as certain components in plants are hydrophilic, which means that they dissolve in water. As such, these elements are preserved in hydrosols but not in essential oils. Hydrosols contain more organic acids, often considered to be anti-inflammatory, as well as other soluble herbal substances. Comparative studies between hydrosols and their essential oils have shown that some are very similar in their chemical make-up, while others are very different. As there are few gas chromatograms (hereafter called GCs) of hydrosols, the chemotypes indicated in the plant descriptions refer to essential oils. However, on the olfactory level we can often detect certain components in hydrosols, such as 1.8 cineol or camphor.

Distillation is not performed in the same way from one producer to another. The length of the distillation, the vapour pressure, the material of the still, and finally the quality of the plant and of the water are key factors affecting the quality of hydrosols, and also the concentration of their active ingredients. It goes without saying that water is probably one of the most important qualitative factors, and that a hydrosol coming from a distillery that uses spring water is not comparable to a product made from stagnant or polluted water.

Furthermore, today it is possible to find producers who make hydrosols exclusively from plants whose essential oils cannot be produced in sufficient volume, such as champaca or jasmine, and these are often of extraordinary quality. For example, in the middle of the Taiwanese jungle I visited a distillery that only makes hydrosols using spring water that flows directly through the still. I have rarely tasted hydrosols of such extraordinary quality.

Aromatic waters have been known for centuries in many cultures. It is difficult to imagine Middle Eastern desserts without rose or orange blossom hydrosol. Known as medicinal waters in China, hydrosols have been used very successfully by therapists, medical doctors and naturopaths in recent years. This success has led producers to supply a wider range of these subtle waters. Today, we can take advantage of the large number of hydrosols which are available internationally.

As with all herbal medicinal products, the result of the therapy depends on the quality of the product. The storage period for a hydrosol is less than that for essential oils. Unfortunately, hydrosols from some suppliers contain preservatives, just as essential oils can be diluted with alcohol or an emulsifier.

Such adulterated products do not have the required quality for the success of hydrosol therapy. Adding essential oils to water does not create a hydrosol. As a hydrosol is acidic, it has a tendency to inhibit the growth of bacteria but not fungi, so hydrosols are not sterile. Certain suppliers expose the hydrosol to an ultra violet ray process in order to prolong its shelf-life. This practice preserves the quality of the hydrosol.

Hydrosols are quite versatile in their use. Their pH of 5–6 makes them particularly appropriate for toning skin, for well-being, for baby care, for use in food recipes and simply for the pleasure of the senses that their use provides. However, I am sure that there are many possibilities that have not been fully explored. I invite you to discover them and use them in your daily lives.

Once upon a time...

In one drop of water are found all the secrets
of all the oceans; in one aspect of You are
found all the aspects of existence.

— *Kahlil Gibran* —

Distilled waters have probably existed for 5000 years, perhaps even longer. One of the most celebrated hydrosols is probably rose water. In 1975, a terracotta vase was discovered in Pakistan which was about 3000 years old, and had been used as a container for rose water. There are many legends and images describing distillation throughout ancient and modern history. Hippocrates (460–c.370 BC, considered to be the 'father of medicine') certainly used hydrosols. There are many historical recipes based on hydrosols:

* In the 14th century, the Queen of Hungary used a medication that contained wine spirits with lemon balm, orange blossom, rose and mint hydrosol.

* At the end of the 14th century, a recipe used by the Carmelites at the Carmes Abbey in Paris adopted lemon balm water as the main ingredient, combined with angelica root, lemon zest, coriander seed, nutmeg, clove and cinnamon. The nuns at the abbey created this famous lemon balm water for centuries.

* Around 1100 BC, the famous Persian doctor Avicenna spoke of aromatic plants distilled for the production of hydrosols, and it appears that he was able to improve the distillation process. Many recipes from this period describing the perfect distillation process still exist to this day.

* In the 18th century, women used hydrosols abundantly both in cooking and for their therapeutic benefits, with some recipes including up to 20 distilled herbs. They sometimes transformed the hydrosol into medication and syrups. Hydrosols were also used in royal courts to perfume and mask body odours. Authors from this period mention up to 200 different hydrosols.

* The Chinese called hydrosols 'medicinal waters', and still use them today in traditional medicine.

* Cleopatra, the famous Egyptian queen, used rose water daily, and boasted of its qualities both for health and for beauty. It is said that rose water was her beauty secret.

* Michelangelo spiced his tea with rose water to calm his explosive character.

* Nonous Theophanous, physician to Emperor Michael of Constantinople, recommended rose water as a remedy for a wide range of problems.

- The Syrian doctor Serration used rose water as an eyewash.

- In the Middle Ages, hydrosols appeared in dispensaries and pharmacies.

- In 1907, the Swiss Pharmacopoeia offered elderberry and linden berry distilled waters.

During the 20th century, interest in essential oils to some extent replaced the use of floral waters and hydrosols, and for many years the lack of commercial interest led to the water from distillation simply being discarded.

However, some hydrosols, such as rose, orange blossom and lavender, have persisted throughout the ages and today hydrosols are once again fully recognised for their benefits and are increasing in popularity.

Energy hydrosol therapy

In the process of falling to the earth, seeping into the ground, and then emerging, water obtains information from various minerals and becomes wise.

— *Masaru Emoto* —

Subtle waters, or hydrosols, are imbued with the soul of the plant. They often act rapidly on psycho-emotional and spiritual levels. It is as if the water was the preferred messenger for the plant. Our body is made up of 70 per cent water and is particularly receptive to the subtle message of plant water. The Japanese researcher Masaru Emoto, known for his book *The Hidden Messages in Water*, showed the extent to which the quality of water can be influenced by sounds and its environment. Hydrosols are the plant's complete imprint. They contain its profound message.

Water embodies elemental power in its pure form. It is vital. Jump into the waves of the ocean, splash your face with water, and you'll feel its regenerative strength. With a hydrosol, we are very close to this vital strength that is, in addition, combined with the healing power of plants. Water is the most common organic link on earth. It is everywhere, both inside and outside our bodies. It is not only the aromatic molecules of hydrosols that determine its properties; water itself is an active ingredient. The ancient Greeks, Egyptians and Romans knew that water had great healing powers, and often considered it a true fountain of youth.

The effectiveness of a hydrosol cannot simply be explained by an intellectual and scientific approach. It would be difficult to imagine that a concentration of aromatic molecules of 2–3 per thousand could be so effective, without taking into account the vibrational dimension of hydrosols. The message that it transmits has a key impact on our physiology.

Plants feed, clothe and protect mankind like a mother. Ancient Ayurvedic medicine teaches us that we need to use the plant in the shape that it reveals itself to us. From an esoteric point of view, the appearance of a large number of hydrosols and essential oils on the international market is probably a blessing from the world of plants to support us and help us heal.

Quality criteria

We remember the quality a long time after the price.

— Gucci —

As I already mentioned, quality is key to therapeutic success. However, it can be difficult for the consumer to make sense of things. One often comes across diluted and polluted hydrosols, and pure, high-quality products are unfortunately hard to find. Given this, here's what we need to consider:

1. Water quality – this is probably one of the most important criteria. It is the living element of the hydrosol: only pure spring water produces quality hydrosols. Unfortunately, many hydrosols are made with sulphated water or water polluted by toxic residues. It is preferable to choose organic or wild plant hydrosols, but this is not a perfect guarantee of quality.

2. The concentration of active ingredients – in contrast to essential oils, the concentration of active ingredients is very low in hydrosols. You'll only find about 2–3 per thousand. However, quality hydrosols will have a higher concentration. To achieve this, it is important that only about the first ten litres of water are collected from the distillation, as after this the hydrosol will have a significantly lower concentration of active ingredients. Olfactory tests are key. Only quality hydrosols have a powerful aroma.

3. One hundred per cent pure and natural – only choose 100 per cent pure hydrosols, if possible from organic or wild plants.

4. Freshness – good-quality hydrosols (i.e. those that have a high concentration of active ingredients) can be stored for 12–24 months, depending on the plant, some even longer. It is preferable to use coloured flasks, as they provide better protection.

5. Price – it goes without saying that a good-quality hydrosol is pricey. Choose specialised suppliers in the field of aromatherapy and herbal medicine. Don't fall for products that appear to be an outstanding bargain, as therapeutic results rely on quality. Prices will vary from one supplier to another. Here as well, it is important to be careful. The price can be ten times higher for a high-quality hydrosol than for a conventional one.

Storage

Pure, natural, good-quality hydrosols can last 12–24 months, sometimes longer. Among the most fragile are elderberry, cornflower, lemon balm and thyme thuyanol. Some hydrosols will last even longer than 24 months. Again, quality is key for the storage period. It is important that the hydrosol has been microfiltered after distillation.

It goes without saying that only bacteriological analysis can determine the level of bacteria in water or in a hydrosol, however, at home an olfactory test can help to find out if the hydrosol is still useable. Spoiled hydrosols no longer have an odour, as the bacteria have destroyed the aromatic particles. The aroma will become sour and acid, somewhat like vinegar.

It is important to avoid exposing hydrosols to light, so store them in coloured flasks and close the flask immediately after use. Glass bottles protect hydrosols from bacteria more effectively than plastic. In hot weather, it is preferable to store hydrosols in the fridge. A temperature of 15–18 degrees is ideal.

Of course, it is necessary to avoid to put your fingers, lips, nose or cotton pads into your hydrosol to prevent the infiltration of bacteria. Oxygen is also an enemy that can degrade the quality of the hydrosol, so it is better to use small vials that have little empty space for everyday use.

Methods of use

There are many ways you can use hydrosols.

- Spray them in the air.

- Use them as a beauty product.

- Use them in the kitchen to improve meals.

And, of course, they are an excellent therapeutic tool.

The main difference between hydrosol therapy and aromatherapy (*even though using hydrosols is part of aromatherapy*) is the fact that hydrosols are easier to use internally and have fewer contraindications. However, specific knowledge is needed to use them properly. Hydrosols can be mixed – a blend of several hydrosols is often more effective than a single one – but it is important to consider the taste because a bad taste can compromise the desire to take the hydrosol properly. Also be careful: by mixing hydrosols you may shorten their shelf-life.

In the kitchen

To preserve their taste and properties only add them at the end of cooking or as a condiment for cold and/or fresh foods as well as desserts. Spray the plates just before serving.

- Hydrosols can add a refined touch to smoothies, fruit juice and fresh vegetables.

- Champaca, kewra, rose, orange blossom and peppermint improve homemade sherbet and ice cream.

- Soft and flowery hydrosols such as rose, champaca, lavender or orange blossom give an exotic note to fruit salads, sherbets and ice cream.

- Spicy hydrosols, such as thyme, savory or basil can make salad dressings taste lighter and less oily.

- Cinnamon, sandalwood or orange blossom hydrosols give a refined taste to chocolate shakes and drinks.

- Stewed meals that can sometimes be heavy seem lighter with a splash of a 'digestive' hydrosol at the end of cooking, such as basil, savory, thyme thymol, cinnamon and rosemary.

- The combinations are limitless for cocktails or shakes.

* Hydrosol ice cubes add a sophisticated note to a cocktail.

For well-being and beauty

A hydrosol is often used in the creation of 'homemade' cosmetics. Even if you don't create your own creams, you can use hydrosols for facial care.

* Hydrosols are excellent tonics, and can be selected according to skin type.

* They can be used for creating clay masks, and also added to existing masks as long as they are made from natural raw material.

* Facial steam baths enriched with hydrosol help to purify the skin and lift blackheads.

* Spraying the whole body with hydrosol after a day at the beach or a hard day at work can reduce stress and enliven the body and mind.

* Regularly spraying the face, including the eyes, with rose, champaca or geranium hydrosol can be beneficial during extended work at the computer.

* Regularly sprinkling the face with soft thyme linalool, palmarosa or lavender hydrosol can help oily or impure skin.

For the air

We are used to dispersing (or diffusing) the scent of essential oils; it is still rather uncommon to spray hydrosols. The aroma of a hydrosol is sometimes softer and more subtle than its corresponding essential oil. Hydrosols are luminous and can have a unique perfume the biochemical components are not always the same as those in essential oils. Certain plants, such as jasmine and champaca, give only an absolute as they provide an insufficient quantity of essential oil. (While essential oils are produced by distillation or pressing, absolutes are obtained by solvent extraction or more traditionally through enfleurage. This way of production is often used for plant material that is too inert for steam distillation, such as jasmine or champaca.) In these cases, the hydrosol is often refined and of very good quality because their producers specialise in hydrosols and rarely, if ever, produce essential oils. Although essential oils and hydrosols don't mix, it is interesting to create hydrosol sprays enriched with essential oils. All you have to do is to shake the bottle before spraying the air.

- Rose hydrosol during a children's birthday party instantaneously calms their over-excitement.

- Jasmine or champaca hydrosol in a bedroom invokes passion.

- Geranium hydrosol in an office creates a positive atmosphere.

- Geranium, peppermint and lavender hydrosol on clothes keep insects away.

- Frankincense hydrosol during a work session enhances communication.

For baby care

Hydrosols are a precious ally to protect and preserve the health of our babies as they are not irritating to fragile skin, are tolerated by babies, and they are effective. They can be added to the bath, on washcloths and also to clean hands. Ingested doses vary depending on age. Internal use can start during the first year, $1/_2$ tsp. (teaspoon) per day in the bottle is enough. Starting at 12 months, 1 tsp. per day.

- Orange blossom or Roman camomile hydrosol in the bottle and in the bath water (1–2 tbsp. (tablespoon)) calms agitated babies. Breastfeeding mothers can spray their nipples with these hydrosols.

- Rose, geranium or lavender hydrosol added to the bath water or in drinks calms babies who are upset.

- Roman camomile hydrosol sprayed on gums calms teething pain (you can dilute the hydrosol half and half with water) and can be used several times a day.

- Roman camomile and basil hydrosol calms colic, and breastfeeding mothers can spray their nipples.

- Lemon verbena and basil hydrosols relieve constipation in babies (in the bottle or sprayed on the nipples).

- In case of a weak immune system, add thyme linalool, palmarosa or frankincense hydrosol to bath water.

- In case of nappy rash, rose, lavender, palmarosa or blue camomile hydrosol can be sprayed locally. (Create a blend or use one of these hydrosols.)

- For rhinitis, a nasal spray with myrtle and/or thyme linalool hydrosol can help.

- To help with insomnia or nightmares, the baby's room can be sprayed with orange blossom and/or champaca hydrosol.

In therapy

The most effective therapeutic use of hydrosols is through ingestion. It is very effective to take a hydrosol as a cure over several weeks, for example during the changing of the season or to reinforce the immune system during an epidemic.

They can generally be taken in a glass of hot water with 1 tbsp. of hydrosol per glass, or 3 times a day in non-sparkling water at room temperature, 1 tbsp. per litre of water. A cure usually takes place over a period of 20–40 days. In this case, you will consume one 200 ml hydrosol bottle every 20 days.

Undeniably, hydrosols have a great purifying effect. They act on the 'energy field' of the individual, and once ingested and absorbed have a direct effect on the whole digestive and metabolic system, whose proper functioning is key to stimulating the immune system defences.

For ingestion

- 1 tsp. in a glass of hot water before or after meals gives 3 opportunities a day to activate the metabolism and support detoxification processes.

- 1 tbsp. in 1 litre of hot or warm water to drink during the day aids metabolic, menopausal or emotional balance problems, and can be beneficial during travel.

- For detox and to fight chronic problems, a period of 40 days is suggested, to be renewed if necessary after a 5-day break.

Externally

- Add a hot or cold compress on the affected area.

- Add to bath water.

- Use in foot baths for painful, bloated or tired feet.

* Use in a sitz bath for urogenital pain, haemorrhoids, genital itching (add 3–5 tsp. to the water).

* Directly spray the affected area.

Gargling or mouthwash

* In case of laryngitis or mouth infection, spray the throat with savory or thyme thymol hydrosol, and/or gargle with the same hydrosols.

* In case of mouth ulcers, wash the mouth with bay laurel hydrosol.

Inhalations

* For rhinitis, bronchitis or sinus infection, inhale thyme thymol, eucalyptus globulus, hyssop officinalis or rosemary verbenon hydrosol. Add 2 tbsp. to a cup of hot water and then inhale.

Enemas

* In case of vaginal infection or candidiasis, rectal or vaginal enemas can be effective. Hydrosols can be diluted in water at a concentration of 20–50 per cent. If you are fasting or doing a detox, you can use an enema with 2 tbsp. of hydrosol in 1 litre of water. Hydrosols are also very useful for colon irrigation.

Nasal spray

* Hydrosol sprays are effective against rhinitis, sinus infection and also for Ayurvedic nasal clearing (neti). Not as well known, but very effective, is the use of hydrosol nasal spray in case of migraines or stiffness, as well as cervical pain.

* In case of a cold (or also allergies), hydrosol-based sprays or a dropper can also be used.

Eye care

* A suitable hydrosol can be used for eyewashes (e.g. myrtle or rose hydrosol) or directly sprayed for tired or burning eyes.

In combination with other herbal medicine approaches

Hydrosols work perfectly with other approaches to herbal medicine.

Aromatherapy

Although hydrosols often present similar benefits to those of essential oils, they are not necessarily identical, even if they come from the same plant and distillation process. The essential oil and its hydrosol contain different biochemical compounds. The water-soluble components are more present in hydrosols, and fat-soluble components are more concentrated in essential oils. The 2 products perfectly complement one another.

Ingesting hydrosols, complemented by the external or olfactory use of essential oils, is often a very effective formula. For prolonged body cleanses and detoxes via ingestion, a hydrosol is definitely more adapted and presents fewer side-effects and contraindications.

Hydrosol therapy is gentler than aromatherapy. This is because of the lower concentration of aromatic molecules. Despite this, experience shows that hydrosols can be particularly effective for alleviating problems relating to the hormonal system. This is why some hydrosols must be avoided during pregnancy, in case of hormone-dependent cancers, and for young children (see indications in the plant descriptions).

Yet even if the concentration of aromatic molecules in hydrosols is minimal, they are often more effective than essential oils for digestive problems, for detoxing, as a metabolic stimulant and as an anti-allergic remedy. Essential oils and hydrosols combine beautifully because they 'come from the same mould'. The combinations can be endless. For example:

- external use of essential oils, combined with ingestion of a hydrosol

- pectoral syrups, a synergy between essential oils and hydrosols

- masks, compresses and so on, mixing essential oils and hydrosols

- essential oils in Fludol or Solubol (*dispersants that dissolve essential oils in water or hydrosols*), used in water with hydrosols.

Gemmotherapy

The mix of hydrosols and gemmotherapy extracts (it is a phytotherapy method which uses plant bud extract and other embryonic plant tissues) is very complementary, and can create very interesting therapeutic synergies. For example:

- raspberry with sandalwood and/or basil for menstrual pain
- birch/cassis with frankincense and/or bay laurel hydrosol for rheumatic pain
- Indian chestnut combined with cypress and/or spikenard for cardiovascular disorders
- olive with angelica hydrosol for nervousness
- hawthorne with orange blossom and spikenard hydrosol for heart rhythm disorders.

Floral elixirs

Hydrosols can be a great base for floral elixirs. For example:

- beech with lavender hydrosol to aid calm judgement and activate tolerance
- plumbago with angelica hydrosol to reinforce decision making
- chicory and rose hydrosol to avoid being too possessive with a loved one.

Herbal teas or concoctions

Hydrosols in this case are added once the tea is made, as it is preferable not to boil them. For example:

- pectoral tea with Scots pine or ravintsara hydrosol
- 'hepatic' tea with rosemary verbenon, ledum, carrot or shiso hydrosol
- 'diuretic' tea with cedar or juniper hydrosol
- green tea with rosemary verbenon, everlasting, juniper or sage hydrosol to stimulate metabolism.

Mother tinctures

Instead of diluting mother tinctures in water, we can dilute them in a hydrosol or a hydrosol mix. For example:

* thyme or hedera mother tincture in eucalyptus hydrosol for an anti-cough drug

* hamamelis, Indian chestnut or red vine mother tincture in cypress hydrosol for venous insufficiency and heavy legs

* gentian or lemon balm mother tincture in coriander hydrosol for digestive problems

* lupulus (hops) mother tincture in rose or orange blossom hydrosol for sleeping problems in children

* crataegus mother tincture in kewra or marjoram hydrosol for cardiovascular problems.

The synergy possibilities with hydrosols are infinite, and an experimental mind can certainly uncover many new possibilities.

Hydrosol therapy for animals

The use of essential oils with pets is rather difficult as some oils that have no contraindications for humans can prove toxic for pets. However, while it can be problematic to use essential oils on animals, do not hesitate to use hydrosols. You can use them to:

* wash infected wounds

* rinse their fur to fight mycosis and other inflammation and infections

* spray irritated eyes – use a gentle hydrosol such as blue camomile

* spray their fur to keep insects and ticks away – lavender and cedar hydrosols

* spray cat fur – spikenard hydrosol is deeply calming, and cats really love the scent

* make compresses for painful joints – sandalwood, cedar and yarrow hydrosols

* prevent and cure fleas – lavender and eucalyptus hydrosols

* spray to calm fear and agitation – orange blossom hydrosol.

Testimonials

'One of my friends has been caring for horses using hydrosols for years now. She noted again and again their effectiveness on wounds, and also for calming this noble animal. Poultices using clay and rose hydrosol often seem to perform miracles on wounds.'

'I was visiting a friend in the South of France. We could see fireworks a long way away. In spite of the distance, her little dog was shaking with fear. I sprayed my friend's hands with orange blossom hydrosol. She rubbed them through its coat. The little dog then licked them, and he immediately calmed down and became still.'

'My thin, apathetic cat was suffering from hyperthyroidism. I added marjoram hydrosol to its drinking water and in 3 days the cat was "back on its feet", had gained weight and was hungry again.'

HYDROSOLS

ANGELICA ROOT – *Angelica archangelica*

Decide with certainty and joy

Portrait of the plant

Angelica is a large aromatic umbelliferous plant, green in colour, which can be found growing wild in rich, moist soil favouring a sunny spot sheltered from the wind.

BOTANICAL FAMILY:	Apiaceous
PART OF THE PLANT DISTILLED:	Roots
TASTE:	Soft, lightly acidic
AROMA:	Woody, sensual

Principal components according to the gas chromatography of the essential oil: monoterpenes

History and mythology

In the Middle Ages, many doctors proclaimed the merits of angelica. They used it to protect themselves from infectious disease and prescribed it as a general tonic during convalescence. Swiss physician Paracelsus fought the plague with angelica root. It is still used as an ingredient in the manufacture of Benedictine and Chartreuse liqueurs. Angelica was used in rituals for divine protection against black magic, witchcraft and diabolical spirits. In Chinese medicine, angelica is one of the main plants used to activate function of the pancreas.

Experiences with angelica root hydrosol

Angelica root hydrosol is indicated for nervous tension and stress-related disorders. It is also very useful for fortifying the system during convalescence. It boosts vitality and protects and strengthens the cardiovascular and immune system. It cleans and detoxifies the body, helping in cases of arthritis, gout, respiratory ailments, flatulence and all kind of digestive problems. We have also observed good results in cases of fibromyalgia, rheumatism and menstrual and back pain. It can be a powerful painkiller in cases of trauma or after surgery.

Energy and psycho-emotional properties

When the pancreas is weakened, the mind becomes tormented, we lack clarity and discernment, and we have trouble making choices and decisions. Angelica hydrosol supports pancreatic function and provides a sense of certainty and serenity. Angelica transmits the strength of Mother Earth, and nourishes Muladhara, the root chakra. As such, it develops a feeling of certainty and assurance. Self-confidence is reinforced, and doubts and fears are allayed. The act of regularly smelling the fragrance of its essential oil combined with a treatment with this hydrosol gives one the necessary courage to make decisions and get rid of doubt. If the air element (the bioenergy described in Ayurveda) is present in excess, we have a tendency to scatter, to doubt, lose our focus and our vision, and we can become anxious. In this case, Angelica hydrosol and its essential oil help us to keep our feet on the ground and stay focused.

Properties and indications

- Spasmolytic, anti-inflammatory and analgesic: menstrual pain and spasm, intestinal cramp, colic, neuralgia, rheumatism, muscular pain

- Digestive, carminative, reduces uric acid, diaphoretic: difficult digestion, flatulence, gastric hyperacidity

- Hepatic and pancreatic stimulant: diabetes, cholesterol, metabolic problems, hypothyroid

- Anti-depressant and depurative: depression, lack of motivation, poor concentration and memory, neurosis, insomnia linked to worry, tormented spirit

- Expectorant: rhinitis, bronchitis

- Immuno-stimulant and general tonic: convalescence, immune system weakness, asthenic states

Suggestions

- When the nerves are frayed, when the mind is anxious, when we have difficulty making decisions, when we lack motivation and vision: undertake a 40-day cure with angelica hydrosol. Take 3 times a day, 1 tsp. in a glass of warm water after meals. Smell the essential oil 3 times a day for 3 minutes, each time with your eyes closed.

- When sleep is difficult because the mind is tormented or anxious: take a bath with 2 tbsp. of angelica hydrosol. Drink a glass of warm water with 1 tbsp. of angelica hydrosol. Rub the soles of your feet with a couple of drops of angelica hydrosol.

- For chronic dry cough, especially in the morning: each morning before eating drink 2 glasses of warm water, each with 1 tsp. of angelica hydrosol, until the symptoms are gone.

- In case of shock: spray the body or the affected area with angelica hydrosol, and repeat every half hour until your nerves have calmed down.

Contraindications

Essential oils are photosensitising. We can't clearly confirm that this is the case with hydrosols. However, some sources do suggest that it is best to avoid using it directly on the skin before exposure to the sun.

BAY LAUREL – *Laurus nobilis*

Develop courage

Portrait of the plant

The laurel is a tree that normally measures 2–6 metres high, but can reach 15 metres. Its branches are straight and grey at the bottom and green at the top. The leaves are lance-shaped, alternating, and tough with ridged sides, and are dark green on the upper surface and lighter on the underside. It gives off an aromatic odour when touched. The whitish flowers are grouped in umbrellas of 4–5 flowers that appear in March or April. It is dioecious: the male and female flowers grow on separate stems. The fruit is a small egg-shaped berry, purplish-black and bare.

BOTANICAL FAMILY:	Lauraceae
PART OF THE PLANT DISTILLED:	Leaves
TASTE:	Spicy, camphor
AROMA:	Characteristic, herbaceous, musky

Principal components according to the gas chromatography of the essential oil: oxides, monoterpenols, monoterpenes

History and mythology

Daphne, the current Greek name of this aromatic plant, evokes its mythological history as the symbol of the Greek god Apollo. According to Ovid, the nymph Daphne was Apollo's first love. She fled from him but was caught after a long chase and at the last minute her father, the river god Pene, transformed her into a laurel. From then on, Apollo made it his favourite tree and consecrated it in victories, songs and poems. The Oracle of Delphi chewed laurel leaves before making prophecies. The Greeks and Romans used laurel as a crown for victors and poets. This tradition continued in the Middle Ages, where bay was used to crown scholars of universities. The famous 'bachelor' degree comes from the Latin *bacca laurea*, which means bay laurel.

Experiences with bay laurel hydrosol

Thanks to its antiseptic and anti-inflammatory properties, it is effective against mouth ulcers and gum inflammation. It acts effectively in cases of inflamed lymphatic ganglions and remains one of the main plants used in treatments for varicose ulcers.

Testimonials

'As a Greek person, I have always been fascinated by the mythologies of my country, and in particular that of the Oracle of Delphi who chewed laurel leaves. One night, before going to bed, I drank a glass of hot water with a tbsp. of this hydrosol. I also dropped a couple of drops of essential oil on my pillow. I had intense dreams all night, as if the plant was talking to me. I received messages concerning therapeutic advice that I could give to people. On waking, the dream was still quite real. Even if my Cartesian side tried to rationalise the experience, a little voice suggested that I remember the message. Later on, I tried to understand it and I discovered aspects of this plant that I had been ignoring, which proved to be very useful. Since then, I've tried to relive the experience from time to time, and my dreams are always intense.'

'A mother came to get help for her daughter who, for several days, had had a mouth full of blisters; so much so that she could no longer eat and was only able to drink with a straw. She took laurel hydrosol internally and by gargling, and very quickly the blisters disappeared. Since then she always makes sure that her daughter has a bottle of bay laurel hydrosol in reserve.'

Energy and psycho-emotional properties

Bay laurel is associated with the throat chakra and the space/ether element. It removes fear, balances emotions, and gives courage and confidence. It transmits a calm strength, and supports psycho-emotional endurance. It's as if it transmits the message that 'everything you need is inside you, now', freeing up the internal power to affirm ourselves and move forward.

Properties and indications

- Bactericidal, virucidal, analgesic, anti-inflammatory: swollen ganglions, mouth ulcers, gingivitis, respiratory disorders, headaches, sprains, epicondylitis

- Digestive, carminative and intestinal antiseptic: bloating, aerophagia, intestinal infections and colds, gastroenteritis, diarrhoea

- Emmenagogue and analgesic: menstrual cramps, amenorrhoea, dysmenorrhoea

- Analgesic, antiseptic, anti-inflammatory, lymphatic and blood stimulant: varicose ulcer, lymphatic and venous stasis

- Fungicide: candidiasis, mycosis, thrush

Suggestions

- In the case of sprains or contusions: use a cold compress (soak a towel in cold water, add 3–6 tbsp. of bay laurel hydrosol) and place on the painful zone. Make hydrosol ice cubes and place them on the wound. (Build up a reserve of ice cubes for children who often injure themselves playing sports.)

- For mouth ulcers, gingivitis or parodontitis, spray the affected area several times a day.

- Mix with geranium and/or palmarosa hydrosol and spray a child's thrush or the treatment zone several times a day.

- Spray varicose ulcers and also drink 2–3 tbsp. of hydrosol a day in water.

- For increased clarity of dreams, drink a cup of hot water with 1 tsp. of bay laurel hydrosol before bed, breathe in the essential oil (apply a couple of drops to your pillow), and spray the hydrosol in the bedroom before going to bed.

- Spray and massage the scalp to treat dandruff, loss of hair and dermatosis (can be mixed with cedar hydrosol).

Culinary advice

❋ Spray boiled potatoes, cabbage and lentils at the end of cooking.

❋ Can replace dried leaves in recipes.

Contraindications

None.

BASIL – *Ocimum basilicum*

Pacify the solar plexus

Portrait of the plant

There are many varieties of basil. This member of the lamiaceae family, originally from India, is one of the rare oriental plants that can be cultivated throughout Europe. There are different *chemotypes* of the essential oil, which means that the biochemistry varies with where it grows. European and Middle Eastern hydrosols are softer, and the main chemotype is linalool. Asian hydrosols are richer in methylchavicol. The following tests and descriptions are based on soft Middle Eastern hydrosols, which nonetheless have a slightly anise nose, indicating the presence of low concentrations of methylchavicol, a very spasmolytic component.

BOTANICAL FAMILY:	Lamiaceae
PART OF THE PLANT DISTILLED:	The whole plant
TASTE:	Soft, spicy
AROMA:	Green, fresh, herbaceous

History and mythology

The name comes from the Greek *basilikos*, meaning 'royal'. This expresses the high value the Greeks gave to this culinary and medicinal plant. They used it as a remedy for vertigo, to reinforce vision, and also for treating respiratory problems. Basil leaves are said to contain magical powers and are used in Africa to protect against bad luck and ward off evil spirits.

Experiences with basil hydrosol

Basil is one of a selection of hydrosols that improve digestion and at the same time calm fragile nerves. It helps women who are nervous, suffering from an excess of *vata*, or during painful periods. A small flask of this hydrosol should be kept with you during flights and can be drunk in warm water, ideally before a meal. It helps protect against motion sickness. Taking 1 ml in a cup of hot water after a heavy meal helps digestion as well as improving hepatic and pancreatic function.

Energy and psycho-emotional properties

Basil hydrosol, drunk in hot water, calms excess symptoms of stress, frayed nerves, mental distraction and an inability to concentrate. It removes discomfort at the solar plexus and transmits a feeling of serenity.

Properties and indications

* Spasmolytic and digestive: colic, spasms, slow and difficult digestion, bloating, flatulence

* Spasmolytic and analgesic: menstrual pain, lumbar, lumbar pain, and a hard and painful abdomen

* Neurotonic: mental agitation, spasms, gastric pain linked to nervousness and mental agitation, migraines linked to stress, and worry, stress, susceptibility

* Slight antihistamine: food intolerance, hay fever

Suggestions

* During the season (when it's cold and dry in winter): drink 1 litre of hot water enriched with 1 tbsp. of basil hydrosol to avoid an increase of *vata* and to protect the nervous system.

* When travelling: carry a small flask of basil hydrosol and drink it in hot or warm water before food (1 tsp. or 20 drops) to improve digestion.

* When studying: drink hot water with basil and rosemary verbenon hydrosol to stay focused and improve memory. At the same time, use essential oils that support concentration, such as tropical basil, lemon, rosemary cineol or rose geranium.

* Blend it with blue camomile hydrosol in cases of hay fever.

- In cases of food intolerance, undertake a 40-day cure, and repeat after a 2-week break if necessary:

  - 1 cup of hot water + 1 tsp. of basil hydrosol before meals, 3 times a day.

  - 1 cup of hot water + 1 tsp. of shiso or ledum hydrosol after meals, 3 times a day.

- If your nerves are frayed and you're confused and unable to concentrate: undertake a 40-day cure with basil hydrosol. Each day, drink 1 litre of water enriched with 1 tbsp. of hydrosol. Smell the essential oil of sweet basil (linalool-type) 3 times a day before meals, eyes closed, for 2 minutes straight.

Culinary advice

- The addition of the hydrosol can replace the fresh plant in tomato sauces and salad dressings when it is out of season.

- Gives a sophisticated note to red fruit desserts (raspberry, strawberry).

Contraindications

None.

BERGAMOT – *Citrus bergamia*

Spark your joy

Portrait of the plant

Bergamot is the fruit of the bergamot tree, from the family rutaceae. According to several sources, it is the result of a cross between bitter orange and lime. The fruit resembles a small orange with greenish flesh and smooth and thick skin. It is yellow on maturity and its flesh is slightly acidic and sour.

BOTANICAL FAMILY:	Rutaceae
PART OF THE PLANT DISTILLED:	Zest
TASTE:	Soft, sour, sharp
AROMA:	Green, fresh, floral, fruity

Principal components according to the gas chromatography of the essential oil: monoterpenes, esters

History and mythology

The legends that explain the presence of bergamot in Southern Italy are varied, with the most likely being that Christopher Columbus imported it from the Canary Islands. Bergamot and petitgrain bergamot essential oils have been used in perfumes for centuries. Bergamot is inedible due to its bitter taste. Only in its homeland, Calabria, is it cooked for hours with sugar to create a type of marmalade. Its perfume has long been an important part of the manufacture of Cologne.

Experiences with bergamot hydrosol

Only recently available, this sparkling and pleasant hydrosol reduces nervous tensions, anxiety and stress. Its sweetness induces feelings of relaxation and joy.

Energy and psycho-emotional properties

This hydrosol helps you feel better about life. It makes life more joyful and prevents you from worrying about problems and existential questions: it shows you when it's time to stop being a slave to physical illusion, to constraints and to manipulation of collective conscious and guilty dependencies. It invites you to transform your bitterness into joy in order to feel better. People who have become cynical, who have lost their openness and innocence, or who have an arrogant attitude can stop taking themselves too seriously.

Properties and indications

* Anti-fungal, virucidal, bactericidal: intestinal infections, respiratory tract infections, fever, acne

* Carminative, digestive, slightly diuretic, hepatic and pancreatic stimulant: bloating, flatulence, hepatic and pancreatic insufficiency, metabolic problems, gastric problems, nausea, heartburn, cramps, constipation

* Stimulates the appetite and digestion: food behaviour problems

* Analgesic: headaches

* Astringent, clarifying, purifying: dermatosis, acne, dilated pores, oily skin

* Anti-stress, anxiolytic, sedative: difficulty going to sleep, stress, mental agitation, hyper-emotional

Suggestions

- During stressful periods: use the hydrosol as an auric spray, and drink a glass of water with 1 tsp. of bergamot hydrosol 2–3 times a day.

- Drink a glass of hot water with 1 tsp. of hydrosol after a heavy meal.

- For nausea or heartburn, directly spray the hydrosol in the mouth and around the body, drink hot water enriched with bergamot hydrosol.

Culinary advice

- Its fresh and fruity taste makes it a great ingredient for fruit-based desserts and cocktails, such as panna cottas, sherbets, fruit juices and smoothies.

- It goes very well with fish.

- It adds great taste to drinking water.

Contraindications

None.

BLUE CAMOMILE – *Matricaria chamomilla*

Become clear and lucid

Portrait of the plant

Blue camomile (also known as German camomile) flowers from May to November and is found growing wild throughout Europe. This single-stem annual plant has a very jagged leaf. The flowers, with white petals and yellow hearts, are brought together in heads, and have a very recognisable aroma.

BOTANICAL FAMILY:	Asteraceae
PART OF THE PLANT DISTILLED:	Flowers
TASTE:	Soft, herbaceous, honey
AROMA:	Soft, enveloping, smoky

Principal components according to the gas chromatography of the essential oil: sesquiterpenes

History and mythology

Camomile is one of the most studied plants and the most used in popular medicine in South Eastern Europe. The botanical name *recutita* means 'truncated' and refers to its very jagged leaves. *Matricaria* signifies 'mother' or 'woman', and can also come from the term 'matrix', referring to the emmenagogue properties of this plant. Ever since antiquity, the matricaria camomile is considered to be a universal anti-inflammatory, analgesic, sedative and digestive remedy. It was also a plant used in gynaecology.

Experiences with blue camomile hydrosol

Various studies confirm again and again the effectiveness of this hydrosol on allergies, whether respiratory or cutaneous, and independent of the allergen. It seems that blue camomile soothes the symptoms. It also soothes inflammation of all sorts: intestinal, urogenital, mouth and so on.

Energy and psycho-emotional properties

Its calming effect makes the mind more lucid and allows one to step back, to free oneself from a defensive attitude and to listen without immediately reacting. Blue camomile hydrosol calms anger and reduces aggressiveness. Calming and sedative, it facilitates sleep after a stressful or agitating day.

Properties and indications

- Neurotonic and calming: works on stress, agitation and anger. It calms when we're ready to 'explode'.

- Analgesic and anti-inflammatory: all kinds of inflammation (cutaneous, urogenital, intestinal in particular); stomach ulcers, colitis, painful menstruation, cutaneous and vaginal itching, inflamed and sore gums, hives, eczema, erythema, wounds

- Antihistaminic: animal hair allergies, hay fever, allergy to the sun, hives, food allergies

- Mucolytic: sinus infection, rhinitis

Suggestions

- Start a cure 4 weeks before the start of hay fever symptoms and continue throughout the season: 1 tbsp. in 1 litre of water to drink during the day: use compresses for irritated eyes, spray the face several times a day.

* In cases of cutaneous eruptions, directly spray the affected zone several times a day, and also drink a cup of hot water with 1 tsp. of blue camomile hydrosol.

* To avoid allergy to the sun: 1 week before departure and during your trip, drink 1 litre of water with 1 tbsp. of this hydrosol, and each night spray the entire body after a shower.

* In case of vaginal itching and inflammation, douche with this hydrosol plus rose and coriander hydrosol.

* For gastric ulcers, drink a cup of hot water with 1 tsp. of blue camomile hydrosol.

* For swollen and inflamed veins, apply as a compress and drink 1 litre of water enriched with 1–2 tbsp. of hydrosol during the day.

* Foot and sitz baths with this hydrosol will have a soothing effect for cramps and painful periods.

Culinary advice

It is particularly useful in drinks at night to help relaxation:

* 1–2 tsp. of hydrosol in warm milk (almond, rice, cow or sheep's milk).

* 1–2 tsp. of hydrosol in a camomile, linden or verbena tea.

Contraindications

None.

ROMAN CAMOMILE – *Chamaemelum nobilis*

Calmly deal with things

Portrait of the plant

This perennial asteraceae grows everywhere in Western Europe on dry, sandy soil rich in silica, and at up to 1000 metres in altitude. Growing to between 10 and 30 cm, its stems are velvety and end with solitary white flower heads. It is also found in North America and Argentina.

BOTANICAL FAMILY:	Asteraceae
PART OF THE PLANT DISTILLED:	Flowers
TASTE:	Soft, honey, sour
AROMA:	Soft, warm, slight note of apple

Principal components according to the gas chromatography of the essential oil: esters

History and mythology

The Egyptians used camomile for its cosmetic effects and as a component for embalming their mummies. Legend has it that Ramses was embalmed with Roman camomile essential oil. The Celts considered it a sacred plant. The Greek name *chamaemelum* comes from the term 'chamos', meaning sand, as it grows close to the ground, and also *melum*, which means apple (referring to its smell, which is similar to this fruit). Roman camomile is named as such because the Romans loved to cultivate this plant.

Experiences with Roman camomile hydrosol

This hydrosol is essential for baby care: impregnate wipes for their buttocks, and spray the breastfeeding mother's nipples or add the hydrosol to the bottle to prevent and soothe colitis. Use as an airspray for baby's room to help them sleep, spray in the mouth during teething, and use in bath water to soften skin and help them relax. Children having tantrums calm down quickly when they are sprayed with this hydrosol. This is a hydrosol you should give as a gift to young mothers.

Furthermore, it also soothes muscular and arterial pain, calms fragile nerves, and fights anxiety and worry. Its calming properties are remarkable.

Testimonial

'A grandmother was able to help her granddaughter get over her fits of anger by spraying her with Roman camomile hydrosol.'

Energy and psycho-emotional properties

From an Ayurvedic perspective, it is an excellent anti-*vata* remedy. It diminishes the bioenergy that creates agitation, pain and difficult digestion. Roman camomile settles the solar plexus and thereby facilitates digestion, whether at the physical or the vibratory level. It helps get over rancour, liberates us from judgement, helps an overly critical mind to step back, and thereby creates the necessary space to open up the heart. Roman camomile hydrosols can also moderate the perfectionist spirit in someone who wants to control everything.

Properties and indications

* Analgesic and anti-inflammatory: colic, gastric pain, menstrual pain, migraines (linked to stress), headaches, intestinal inflammation, gastric ulcers

* Spasmolytic: intestinal spasms, gastric pain, newborn colic

* Calming and anti-inflammatory: inflammation of the eyes (also for babies), styes, conjunctivitis

* Irritated, sensitive, reddened skin

Suggestions

* For babies who suffer during teething, spray the hydrosol several times a day in the buccal cavity, massage their cheeks 1–2 times a day with 1 drop of essential oil.

* With newborn colic, add 1 tsp. of hydrosol twice a day to the bottle, or directly spray the breastfeeding mother's nipples.

* For a perfectionist mind with a need to control everything and a lack of serenity, undertake a 40-day cure with 1 tbsp. of hydrosol in 1 litre of still water to drink during the day.

Culinary advice

* Excellent nighttime tea that promotes relaxation and sleep:

  – 1–2 tsp. of hydrosol in warm milk (almond, rice, cow or sheep milk)

  – 1–2 tsp. of hydrosol in camomile, linden or verbena tea.

Contraindications

None.

CARROT SEED – *Daucus carota*

Transmit a feeling of security

Portrait of the plant

Daucus carota is the wild ancestor of the domestic carrot and a common wildflower found in dry fields, roadside ditches and open areas. This plant is easy to grow from seed and performs best in well-drained to dry soils, with low to moderate soil fertility. The carrot is widespread in the wild. It doesn't grow well in high altitudes, but flourishes in both warm and cold climates.

BOTANICAL FAMILY:	Umbelliferae
PART OF THE PLANT DISTILLED:	Seeds
TASTE:	Earthy and a bit spicy and acidic, stays for a long time in the mouth
AROMA:	Woody, soft, comforting

Principal components according to the gas chromatography of the essential oil: sesquiterpenols

History and mythology

This vegetable has been cultivated for over 2000 years and has become very popular in kitchens around the world. For many of us, the carrot is probably the first solid vegetable that we ate. This plant represents not only an important food but is also used for remedies, and is traditionally known for the warming qualities of its seeds and leaves. The botanical name *Daucus* comes from the Greek *daio*, which signifies 'warm myself'. In ancient Greece, the doctors suggested concoctions made from carrot seeds for problems of cooling of the urinary tract and for all other problems linked to the 'cold', such as coughs and colds. It was also suggested for liver, pancreas and spleen degeneration.

Experiences with wild carrot hydrosol

This hydrosol often works well for hepatic regeneration. After a cure with carrot hydrosol, cholesterol rates often come back to normal. At the cutaneous level, the hydrosol is regenerative and helps tired skin to recuperate faster, especially after a long illness or intense medical treatment.

Energy and psycho-emotional properties

Like its essential oil, the hydrosol transmits a feeling of security and protection at the psycho-emotional level. It is especially useful for people who are scatter-brained, stressed and hypersensitive, with an excess *vata*. It fights susceptibility and nervous fragility, and helps one become more certain without adopting a defensive attitude.

Properties and indications

* Depurative and regenerating for liver, kidneys and pancreas, blood purifier: cholesterol, diabetes, weak metabolism, water retention, obesity, hepatitis

* Cardiovascular regulator: venous stasis, venous weaknesses, varicose veins, haemorrhoids

* Cutaneous and cell regeneration, anti-ageing effect on the skin: eczema, dermatosis, aged and damaged skin, wrinkles, scars, irritated skin, rosacea

* Neurotonic: particularly useful for nervous people who lack confidence

Suggestions

* Undertake a cure in spring time (the cold and wet season corresponds to *kapha* bioenergy), combined with rosemary verbenon hydrosol, to

regenerate hepatic functions and activate metabolism. For 40 days, take 1–2 tbsp. of hydrosol in 1 litre of water during each day.

❀ Avoid cures during the summer, as this hydrosol is quite warming. However, it can be useful after a holiday on the beach to spray the skin before applying natural oils or creams. This will support cutaneous firming.

❀ It combines well with other metabolism depurative and stimulating hydrosols, such as helichrysum, ledum, rosemary verbenon and shiso.

❀ People who always need to be reassured can undertake the 40-day cure (see above) and use the hydrosol as an auric spray, misting it around themselves several times a day.

Culinary advice

Adding it at the end of cooking gives soups an acidic and musky taste.

Contraindications

Pregnancy; avoid skin contact before exposure to the sun.

Atlas cedar (wood) – *Cedrus atlantica*

See the goal, think big

Portrait of the plant

These majestic coniferous trees can rise to a height of 40 metres, reach 100 years of age and grow at altitudes up to 2000 metres. The cedar is powerful and has an 'unalterable' quality as its wood contains a strong percentage of essential oils that parasites, bacteria and moulds cannot attack. It is very durable and keeps insects and bad spirits away.

Botanical family:	Coniferous, pinacea
Part of the plant distilled:	Wood
Taste:	Sour, astringent
Aroma:	Woody, resinous, soft, hot

Principal components according to the gas chromatography of the essential oil: sesquiterpenes

History and mythology

In biblical times, cedar symbolised strength, spiritual greatness, dignity, the aristocracy and courage. The term 'cedrus' comes from the Arab word *kieron*, which means strength. Cedar is thus *the* symbol for incorruptibility and immortality. In the 2nd century, the philosopher Origen wrote, 'Cedar does not wither; using cedar for the beams of our houses protects the soul from corruption', and for centuries ancient civilisations in the Middle East built their ships, palaces and furniture with Lebanese cedar wood.

Experiences with atlas cedar hydrosol

This hydrosol helps people who lack confidence and objectivity in their lives. It soothes heavy legs, varicose veins and haemorrhoids. It revitalises and detoxifies hair in cases of dandruff, loss of hair or itching.

Energy and psycho-emotional properties

This hydrosol fights hypersensitivity and nervous fragility and helps us to affirm ourselves without adopting a defensive attitude. It is clear that people who use this hydrosol increase their dignity and self-respect and establish a better relationship with their physical body.

Properties and indications

- Analgesic: sciatic nerve, rheumatism, lumbago, migraine, arthritis

- Anti-asthmatic: it helps people who suffer from asthma attacks, especially if psychosomatic or provoked by stress

- Cardiotonic, lymphatic activator, arterial regenerator, lymphatic and venous decongestant: excellent for pain in the cardiac region, tachycardia, heavy legs, cellulite, swelling, venous stasis, atherosclerosis, haemorrhoids, varicose veins, congestion in the area of the hips

- Depurative, anti-parasite, litholytic: intestinal parasites and mycosis, diabetes, kidney stones

- Healing, cutaneous astringent and regenerator: wounds, varicose ulcers, hives, dermatosis and itchy scalp, loss of hair, cutaneous allergic reactions, sensitive skin, rosacea

- Neurotonic: lack of motivation and goals

Suggestions

- For loss of hair, itchiness, dandruff, scalp dermatosis, undertake a 21-day cure: spray the scalp and massage it with the hydrosol on dry hair. It can be combined with sage or rosemary verbenon hydrosols. For loss of hair, combine with lavender and spikenard hydrosols. For itchiness, combine with rose, coriander or lavender hydrosols.

* Cellulite, circulatory troubles and heavy legs: combine with other circulatory hydrosols based on the psycho-emotional profile of the person, such as cypress, sandalwood, yarrow, spikenard, kewra, myrtle, Scots pine, everlasting or vetiver. A foot bath with cedar hydrosol soothes heavy legs.

* For eczema, acne or itchiness, spray the affected zone or use compresses.

* As its nose is rather masculine and woody, men can use it as a tonic. It is a soothing aftershave, and it is astringent and antiseptic. In cases of rosacea or acne, spray the face several times a day.

* For lack of objectivity, motivation and confidence, or being fearful about the future, undertake a 40-day cure: 1 tbsp. in 1 litre of water to drink during the day. Use the hydrosol as an auric spray. Additionally, apply a drop of its essential oil each morning to the top of the scalp near the crown chakra and around the cervical area.

* Spray the cedar hydrosol on dog, cat and horse coats to protect against insects and ticks (dogs seem to like the smell of this hydrosol). The hydrosol seems also to be effective in certain cases of dermatosis in cats.

Culinary advice

Sophisticated and surprising: 1 tsp. in 1 glass of grape juice.

Contraindications

Even if the risks are minimal, you should probably avoid this hydrosol during pregnancy and with children under 5. Physical risks are unlikely, but with regards to energy it is not a plant to use during these periods of life.

CHAMPACA – *Michelia champaca or Michelia alba*

Enchant the heart

Portrait of the plant

This magnoliaceae is a large tree that can grow up to 50 metres high and is cultivated not only for its wood but also as a decorative shrub for its very perfumed flowers. It gives off an intoxicating odour of vanilla and is very sensual – qualities that are clearly found in its hydrosol.

BOTANICAL FAMILY:	Magnoliaceae
PART OF THE PLANT DISTILLED:	Flowers
TASTE:	Soft, floral, sensual, vanilla
AROMA:	Floral, sensual, suave, intoxicating

History and mythology

In India, champaca is a mythological flower which finds mention in numerous legends. One of its names in Sanskrit, Nag Champa, makes reference to Nagar, the Serpent god, as its petals resemble a snake's head. These flowers are often used for the creation of frankincense sticks and during pujas, or spiritual ceremonies. Newlyweds' beds are decorated with champaca and jasmine. Champaca also symbolises reincarnation, eternal life and the dissolution of illusion that death represents. It is also the link between Vishnu and Shiva, the freeing of the self, and the victory of joy over the ego.

Experiences with champaca hydrosol

Its very seductive scent makes this hydrosol an excellent ambiance spray. It encourages deep relaxation and is probably one of the most helpful hydrosols for shutting out daily life and opening oneself to sensual experiences. Its exquisite and sensual taste is greatly appreciated and it is a great culinary addition to desserts. It is definitely an aphrodisiac through its fragrance and taste. It balances the *pitta* bioenergy, diminishes gastric acidity, helps control cravings and the excessive need for sugar, and calms people who eat due to frustration or stress.

Energy and psycho-emotional properties

Champaca can be used for lack of sexual desire, emotional indifference and a lack of understanding of the meaning of life. If meeting up with someone you love leaves you feeling indifferent, champaca can help you open up your heart to once again feel joy. It has remarkable benefits for energy, both ingested and as an ambiance spray. Sprayed on the skin, it envelops you in softness. It is an ideal remedy for frustration, dissatisfaction, exaggerated expectations and anger. It calms people who overreact. It balances feminine and masculine aspects.

Properties and indications

- Analgesic and anti-inflammatory at the digestive level: nausea, vomiting, ulcers, gastric acidity, bulimia, cravings, diarrhoea, abdominal pain

- Analgesic and anti-inflammatory at the muscular and articular level: rheumatism, migraines, arthritis

- Healing, cutaneous regeneration, astringent, anti-inflammatory: varicose ulcers, wounds, rosacea

- Nervous system and cardiac tonic: palpitations, agitation, anger, neurasthenia

- Aphrodisiac: sexual indifference, frigidity, dysfunction

Suggestions

※ For depression, sexual and emotional indifference, or frustration, undertake a 40-day cure: drink 1 litre of water with 1 tbsp. of this hydrosol and regularly spray the face and aura. It is also useful during heatwaves to freshen the air.

※ For excessive appetite, bulimia or gastric acidity, drink a cup of hot water with 1 tsp. of this hydrosol before meals. Also drink a cup of hot water with 1 tsp. of the hydrosol in case of excessive appetite. In this case, it can also be combined with sandalwood, coriander, kewra and rose hydrosols.

Culinary advice

This is one of my favourite hydrosols for its taste, as it:

※ gives a sophisticated taste to fruit-based desserts

※ gives a soft flowery and vanilla note to smoothies, fruit juices and lhassi

※ improves the taste of water, making it floral, soft and suave.

Serve water enriched with champaca hydrosol with hot and spicy meals in order to avoid excess *pitta* and heartburn.

Contraindications

None.

Cinnamon bark – *Cinnamomum verum*

Break the ice

Portrait of the plant

The cinnamon tree grows to a height of 10–15 metres with green leaves and greenish flowers. Its fruits are small berries, purple in colour. The bark is harvested during the rainy season and rolled up, creating the famous sticks. Part of the laurel family, it grows in tropical zones.

BOTANICAL FAMILY:	Lauraceae
PART OF THE PLANT DISTILLED:	Bark
TASTE:	Spicy, sour, soft
AROMA:	Hot, woody, soft, powdery

Principal components according to the gas chromatography of the essential oil: aromatic aldehydes

History and mythology

This famous spice has been used since antiquity and is a component in many traditional pharmaceutical preparations. It is used as an ingredient in spiritual ceremonies and also as a culinary spice. The Egyptians used it for embalming and as a perfume, in the same way as frankincense, and also for cooking. Chinese medicine counts cinnamon as one of the 50 main medicinal plants and considers it a great energy regenerator, even mentioning that it can bring on immortality. Ayurveda teaches us that cinnamon purifies *Raktadhatus*, meaning the blood.

Experiences with cinnamon hydrosol

A 40-day cure (1–2 tbsp. of hydrosol in 1 litre of water to drink during the day) can reduce triglycerides, glucose and cholesterol levels by 25–30 per cent. Combined with angelica hydrosol, it increases dynamism and transmits courage and strength during healing. It stimulates sexual appetite and 'breaks the ice'. We may notice that overly critical people express more enthusiasm and passion, and become less perfectionist after a cure with this hydrosol. Its warmth helps those scared of love, those who don't dare. It is also effective in cases of chronic cystitis and other urogenital inflammation and infection.

Testimonial

'A 40-day cure with this hydrosol helps introverted and timid people better express themselves and feel more connected with others.'

Energy and psycho-emotional properties

Cinnamon hydrosol fortifies the nervous system, warms the heart and reinforces motivation and dynamism. It reduces the fear that makes us feel distant and cold, and breaks down the walls the ego builds to protect itself. It helps us become less isolated and overcomes the mistrust caused by deception. In this way, it creates the space necessary to be able to live relationships with passion, creativity and enthusiasm.

Properties and indications

* Anti-inflammatory and analgesic: rheumatism, dental pain, migraines

* Antibacterial: respiratory tract and urogenital infections

* Metabolic stimulant: hepatic and pancreatic insufficiency, diabetes, cholesterol, obesity

* Immune system stimulant: colds, asthenia

* Digestive and antiseptic: diarrhoea, vomiting, bad breath, colic, buccal infections

* Cardiotonic: cardiac weakness, shortness of breath

* Diuretic, uterotonic, aphrodisiac: dysmenorrhoea, amenorrhoea, childbirth, urinary infections, libido problems

Suggestions

- In cases of fatigue or in busy periods during studies or exams, drink 1 glass of hot water with 1 tsp. of cinnamon hydrosol 3 times a day.

- For bad breath, drink 1 litre of flat water enriched with 1 tbsp. of hydrosol per day, and use as a mouthwash and for gargling.

- For diarrhoea, drink a cup of hot water with 1 tsp. of cinnamon hydrosol 3–5 times a day.

- For a lack of enthusiasm or passion, or sexual frigidity, drink a cup of hot water with 1 tsp. of cinnamon hydrosol twice a day, smell the cinnamon essential oil 3 times a day for 2 minutes straight, eyes closed. Also, spray the hydrosol on the stomach and lower back before sex, and use it as an ambiance spray in the bedroom.

Culinary advice

The cinnamon is known worldwide for its taste.

- Spicy and delicious in fruit sauces, marmalades and apple desserts.

- Gives a warm and spicy smell to black teas and makes them more digestible.

- Delicious in apple juice.

- Gives character to fruit juice cocktails and is revigorating.

Contraindications

Uterotonic – avoid during pregnancy.

CISTUS – *Cistus ladaniferus*

Heal wounds from the past

Portrait of the plant

Cistus ladaniferus is a shrub that grows in most Mediterranean countries. The difference between the cistus ladaniferus compared with other cistaceae is that it secretes a gum during the summer to protect it from the strong heat. It varies in height from 30 cm to 1 metre. Its flowers are made up of 5 petals and only last for a day.

BOTANICAL FAMILY:	Cistaceae
PART OF THE PLANT DISTILLED:	Leaves
TASTE:	Hot, smoky, astringent
AROMA:	Musky, balsamic

Principal components according to the gas chromatography of the essential oil: monoterpenes, monoterpenols, esters

History and mythology

The Egyptians and Hebrews used cistus ceremonially. It was an integral part of rituals to connect with the spiritual self and become conscious of the shadow and mechanisms used by the occult. Its merits for spiritual purification were proclaimed.

Experiences with cistus hydrosol

It is often effective in slowing down internal haemorrhages in the case of fibroids, haemorrhagic ulcers and haemorrhagic periods, or also to avoid post-operation bleeding. Excellent for washing bleeding wounds, it is astringent, healing and regenerative at the cutaneous level.

Testimonials

'One day my dog was brutally attacked by another, and I quickly took it to the vet for stitches. When I picked it up that evening it was depressed. I made a mix of everlasting hydrosol and cistus hydrosol and gave it orally with a bit of water. Two hours later, its outlook had changed and its joy of life had returned.'

'Following a removal of a cyst in her breast, one of my patients was worried because the scar would not heal and continued to ooze. As she refused to use essential oils, I suggested a cistus hydrosol in a compress, and in 1 day the wound had closed.'

Energy and psycho-emotional properties

Whether with its essential oil or hydrosol, cistus is a plant that helps us recognise the origin of the mechanisms that force us always to react in the same way to obstacles. One has to imagine that at the level of our subtle bodies, there can be wounds that continue to 'bleed' and ensure that, despite the effort and work that we do, we continue to adopt the same mental and psycho-emotional behaviour. Cistus works deeply on the source of the problem, bypassing the mental block. It is effective even if we are not aware of it, and it can dissolve deep blockages. It is interesting to undertake a 40-day cure with cistus hydrosol, combining it with shiso hydrosol (see suggestions).

Properties and indications

* Powerful bactericide and virucidal, stimulates the immune system: chronic cough and bronchitis, auto-immune illnesses, herpes, chicken pox, measles, dermatosis

- Haemostatic, astringent and antiseptic: bleeding wounds, nosebleeds, uterine bleeding, fibroids, endometriosis, recto-colic haemorrhaging, Crohn's disease, haemorrhagic periods

- Astringent, firming, healing: acne, asphyxiated skin, wrinkles, dilated pores, shaving cuts

- Neurotonic: stress, self-destructive behaviour

Suggestions

- If you want to change your mental behaviour, every morning, drink a cup of hot water with 1 tsp. of shiso hydrosol and massage the pancreas zone with a couple of drops of this essential oil. In the afternoon, drink a cup of hot water with 1 tsp. of shiso hydrosol. Before going to bed, drink a cup of hot water with 1 tsp. of cistus hydrosol. Apply one drop of cistus essential oil between the upper lip and nose and also on the third eye. Say the word *revelation* 7 times before sleeping.

- For endometriosis and haemorrhagic periods, 7 days before your period starts, drink 1 litre of water per day enriched with 2 tbsp. of cistus hydrosol. Continue during your period until the bleeding stops.

- If you often tend to talk about the same thing during work meetings, and have difficulty being authentic with colleagues, spray the meeting room with this hydrosol before the meeting.

Contraindications

None.

CLARY SAGE – *Salvia sclarea*

Inspiration and creativity

Portrait of the plant

This is a biennial herbaceous plant with a short life, which is very odorous and velvety and can grow from 40 cm to 100 cm. Its leaves are large, oval-shaped and rough. The flowers are pink, lilac and pale blue and about 3 cm across.

BOTANICAL FAMILY:	Lamiaceae
PART OF THE PLANT DISTILLED:	Whole plant
TASTE:	Soft, astringent, spicy
AROMA:	Musky, floral, spicy

Principal components according to the gas chromatography of the essential oil: esters

History and mythology

It was called 'clear eye' in the Middle Ages as it supposedly had an important role in eye treatments. Furthermore, shamans, priests, alchemists and healers from numerous European and Asian cultures thought that the perfume of clary sage increased visionary capacity and helped to distinguish between good and evil.

Experiences with clary sage hydrosol

Known for its help in regulating the menstrual cycle, this hydrosol is also excellent for improving morale and zest for life. I have often been able to observe that it helps women suffering from premenstrual symptoms, acting on pain, bloating, water retention and the lack of emotional control.

Testimonial

'I lacked motivation and was going through a passive phase, lacking vision and a clear goal. My therapist suggested I undertake a 40-day cure by blending clary sage hydrosol with lemon verbena, taking it in the morning in a glass of hot water with 1 tsp. of clary sage hydrosol, and at night with a glass of hot water and 1 tsp. of lemon verbena. I also used the 2 hydrosols as auric and air sprays. One week later my emotional state had completely changed, I was full of ideas and I wanted to take my life in my own hands. I subsequently moved and changed jobs. Ever since then these 2 hydrosols have been my companions whenever my morale is low.'

Energy and psycho-emotional properties

Clary sage supports us when we have psychic problems. It dissolves deep tension at the same time as being both revitalising and stimulating. It is a very effective remedy for fear, depression and paranoia. It has a long-term calming effect, and removes melancholy thanks to its revitalising effect. Like its essential oil, the hydrosol is associated with the throat chakra, creating the necessary space for creativity and making one euphoric and enthusiastic. Spraying this hydrosol in the bedroom before sleep helps us to perceive dreams with greater clarity. Clary sage is a plant for creative people as it opens them up to the unknown and brings new inspiration.

Properties and indications

* Oestrogen-like, antispasmodic, anti-inflammatory: premenstrual syndrome, oligomenorrhoea, dysmenorrhoea, period pain, hot flashes, low morale linked to hormonal imbalance

* Euphoria-inducing, anxiolytic, anti-depressant, a nervous system balancer: phobia, fears, depression

* Anti-stress: helps to stay balanced during periods of heavy workload and change

Suggestions

* If you have recently stopped taking the birth control pill and it is taking your body a little time to regain its natural balance (e.g. regular periods), undertake a 40-day cure taking 1 tbsp. of clary sage hydrosol in 1 litre of hot water every day.

- ✦ Spray the air and around the body to stimulate creativity but also to get rid of pessimism and gloom.

- ✦ Apply a hot compress to the stomach in case of cramps and abdominal pain during periods.

- ✦ Add to a clay mask when acne-like pimples appear before periods.

- ✦ Spray the air and the mouth in case of stress.

- ✦ Use in combination with yarrow hydrosol in order to better accept life changes.

Culinary advice

Surprising and interesting in desserts and fruit juices.

Contraindications

Pregnancy, mastosis or hormone-dependent cancer.

CORIANDER – *Coriandrum sativum*

Calm the fire to see the truth

Portrait of the plant

This is an aromatic plant that is cultivated in temperate zones around the world, and is used in many culinary dishes. It is also called Arab or Chinese parsley. The name coriander comes from the Greek *koriannon* or Latin *coriandrum*. The name *korion* is also mentioned in Mycenaean tables, and also *koris*, which signifies bed bugs, probably alluding to the similarity between the plant's seeds and the insect. Coriander is probably originally from the Eastern Mediterranean region. In Latin America and in certain Caribbean countries it is called cilantro.

BOTANICAL FAMILY:	Apiaceae
PART OF THE PLANT DISTILLED:	Seeds
TASTE:	Astringent, sour, soft, spicy
AROMA:	Fresh, rosy, soft, spicy

Principal components according to the gas chromatography of the essential oil: monoterpenols

History and mythology

The Egyptians said that coriander is a plant that makes you happy, and they used it as an aphrodisiac. Mentioned in *One Thousand and One Nights,* in the Orient it was used as an aphrodisiac. The Chinese said it had virtues for immortality and digestive properties. Ayurvedic medicine uses it as a major remedy for calming excess *pitta*, meaning an excess of the fire element. Hippocrates used coriander to treat stomach spasms. It was the Romans who introduced it to Western Europe.

Experiences with coriander hydrosol

Coriander hydrosol is effective when the digestive fire is too high, causing bad breath, excessive thirst and a constant feeling of being bloated. It calms the fire both at the physical and psycho-emotional level, which allows one to be more serene and less 'inflamed'. It supports pancreatic function and also calms muscular pain.

Energy and psycho-emotional properties

Coriander calms the fire. It soothes extreme emotions and allows one to be more authentic and serene. As such, it creates the necessary space for us to act without being emotional, to see the truth, and develop creativity. It helps us to evolve, calmly affirming our self, and concentrate on the job at hand.

Properties and indications

* Neurotonic and analgesic: mental confusion, weak memory, difficulty with concentration, vertigo, irritability, anger, aggressive attitude, susceptibility, migraines, dental pain

* Anti-inflammatory and decongestant at the respiratory level: smoker's cough, hoarseness, chronic bronchitis

* Antispasmodic and anti-inflammatory at the muscular level: soreness and cramps linked to sports

* Cardiotonic and blood purifier: haemorrhoids, varicose veins, venous inflammations, alcoholism

* Powerful bactericide and virucide, reinforces the immune system: chronic cough and bronchitis, auto-immune illnesses, herpes, chicken pox, measles, dermatosis

* Anti-inflammatory and diuretic: prostate inflammation, chronic cystitis

* Digestive fire balancer and depurative: diabetes, excessive thirst (sometimes due to too much alcohol), bloated abdomen, diarrhoea, colic, bad breath, strong and malodorous transpiration, stomach ulcers, craving, excessive appetite

- Anti-inflammatory at the level of the eyes: eye inflammation (excess *pitta*), conjunctivitis

- Healing, bactericide, soothing: ulcers, acne, hives

Suggestions

- Take a 40-day cure with coriander hydrosol: 2 tbsp. in 1 litre of water every day, and eliminate alcohol and other drugs. This cure is also recommended for lack of clarity and ocular weakness.

- Use as a mouthwash in case of bad breath, and regularly spray the buccal cavity with this hydrosol.

- Use as a compress for eye inflammation.

- *Pitta*-type people can regularly consume this hydrosol during the hot season in order to be less controlled by their emotions and to balance excessive appetite, for example: 1 glass of water or a cup of hot water with 1 tsp. of hydrosol before meals.

Culinary advice

- A broth enriched with sandalwood and coriander hydrosols served before the meal helps to digest heavy meals and to feel more satisfied.

- Add 1 tbsp. to curry at the end of cooking.

- Spray a salad.

- Adding it to a gazpacho can reinforce the refreshing effect.

- Add it to an Indian raita or a Greek tzatziki (yogurt with cubed vegetables, such as cucumbers, tomatoes and onions).

Contraindications

None.

Cypress – *Cupressus sempervirens*

Go towards the essence

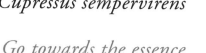

Portrait of the plant

Cypress belongs to the coniferous family, and is found throughout the northern hemisphere. This tall, slender tree can grow 20–30 metres high. The cypress, representative of the Mediterranean flora, is also the tree of cemeteries and a symbol of grieving in southern countries. Its longevity and its persistent foliage are excellent symbols of immortality. The Latin name *sempervirens* means 'ever green'.

Botanical family:	Coniferous
Part of the plant distilled:	Shoots
Taste:	Spicy, astringent
Aroma:	Woody, amber, camphor, tonic

Principal components according to the gas chromatography of the essential oil: monoterpenes

History and mythology

Greek mythology dedicates the cypress to Pluto, god of the dead, and describes this tree as the image of eternity. This conifer has become a symbol of grieving, of eternal life and resurrection, but also of psychological transformation. It is found in most cemeteries around the Mediterranean Sea. In China, the cypress is also seen as a symbol of immortality. They say that consuming cypress seeds prolongs life.

Experiences with cypress hydrosol

Cypress hydrosol is excellent as a venous and lymphatic decongestant. It is often used, along with its essential oil, in the treatment of circulatory problems such as venous stasis, varicose veins, haemorrhoids and cellulite, and as a tonic in cases of rosacea. It is also a main ingredient in cough syrups, and a metabolic stimulant. It helps us to remain focused on specific objectives.

Energy and psycho-emotional properties

The cypress is synonymous with immortality of the soul. Its message of moderation and virtue tells us to take our time in existential reality. It helps control excesses and wasting of energy, supports self-control and channels energy, and focuses our concentration on what is important. As a symbol of eternity, it reminds us that death is not the end but a new beginning. It reinforces the nervous system, helps us resist temptations and to remain clear and concentrated. It supports people drowning in their emotions. It allows bed-wetting children and incontinent people to increase their bladder control.

Properties and indications

* Stimulates pancreatic, hepatic and kidney functions: depurative, oedema, gout, arthrosis, cystitis, slow metabolism, obesity

* Circulatory stimulant, venous decongestant: cellulite, varicose veins, haemorrhoids, rosacea, heavy legs

* Pelvis decongestant: premenstrual syndrome, lumbar and premenstrual pain, prostate inflammation, urinary infections

* Anti-cough: bronchitis, cough

* Enuresis, incontinence

* Astringent at the cutaneous level: flabby skin, cellulite, rosacea, itching

* Hormonal balancer: menopause, premenopausal, hot flashes, excessive sweating

Suggestions

* Haemorrhoids: combine with yarrow, sandalwood, cistus, everlasting, spikenard or vetiver hydrosols (based on the psychological profile of the person). Take internally and via sitz baths. Then apply an aromatherapeutic blend.

* For varicose veins, cellulite and purplish skin, take internally and use compresses on the indicated zone (by combining the same hydrosols for haemorrhoids). Then apply an aromatherapeutic mix.

* For premenstrual pain, use a warm compress. Soak a towel in hot water, add 2–3 tbsp. of hydrosol and place on the affected zone.

* In the case of prostatitis or cystitis, undertake a 40-day cure by combining it with yarrow, sandalwood, cedar, juniper and peppermint hydrosols. Drink 3–4 times a day in a cup of hot water with one of these hydrosols or with a mix. Use a hot compress to alleviate congestion in the pelvis.

* For urinary tract infections, use in combination with cinnamon, coriander and sandalwood hydrosol.

Contraindications

Mastosis, hormone-dependent cancer.

Eucalyptus globulus

Pacify the mind

Portrait of the plant

The eucalyptus is originally from Australia and Tasmania, and today also grows in Mediterranean countries and in California. It can grow up to 50 metres in height, and is characterised by large pointed leaves, grey-green in colour and full of odour, and small white flowers covered by a sort of membrane. Some 700 different eucalyptus species are known to exist, with 500 producing essential oils!

BOTANICAL FAMILY:	Myrtaceae
PART OF THE PLANT DISTILLED:	Leaves
TASTE:	Astringent, fresh
AROMA:	Aromatic, camphor, a bit foul

Principal components according to the gas chromatography of the essential oil: oxides

History and mythology

Australian aboriginals used this tree for different medical purposes. English settlers adopted some of these recipes and added their own knowledge. Until the end of the 19th century, eucalyptus was planted widely in subtropical regions in order to dry up swampy zones. As a result of these plantations, tropical fevers, in particular malaria, were able to be eradicated. In certain regions of Italy, they continue to speak of the eucalyptus as a 'fever tree'. Its name comes from the Greek *kalypto* which means cover, probably alluding to the form of its flower.

Experiences with eucalyptus globulus hydrosol

Known for its respiratory properties, it also heals oily skin and acne. As it helps assimilate oxygen, it can be used for asthenia (general debility), and it transmits clarity and also activates the thyroid. Ocular compresses heal styes and conjunctivitis.

Energy and psycho-emotional properties

This powerful plant teaches the ability to survive. As it is able to dry swampy land, it also drains our 'internal swamps', dissolves internal conflicts, helps us to see clearly and be aware of reality as it is. Eucalyptus opens our eyes to the world. If we are drowning in emotions, it is difficult to remain objective and realistic. Eucalyptus clarifies ideas, helps concentration, and stimulates and transmits the necessary energy we need to act in an appropriate way.

Properties and indications

* Mucolytic and expectorant: rhinitis, sinusitis, bronchitis, colds

* Anti-diabetic and thyroid stimulant, hepatorenal and pancreatic stimulant: diabetes, slow metabolism, water retention, obesity, chronic fatigue, hypothyroidism

* Antioxidant and antiseptic: acne, infectious dermatitis, styes, conjunctivitis, eye irritations

* Depurative and draining: diabetes, cholesterol

* Cessation of smoking

Suggestions

* Stopping smoking, lack of clarity, inability to see reality for what it is, lack of intuition: undertake a 40-day cure with 1 tbsp. of hydrosol in 1 litre of water to drink during each day.

* For styes, conjunctivitis or irritated eyes, use eye compresses.

* Make a nasal spray for rhinitis, sinusitis or nasopharyngitis (recipes given later in this book).

* Use in a clay mask, as a compress or facial sauna in cases of acne.

Culinary advice

◉ Use to make warming and preventative teas in case of cold pandemics.

Contraindications

None.

Everlasting – *Helichrysum italicum*

Discover the hidden charges of the past

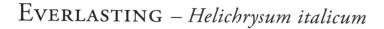

Portrait of the plant

A perennial and very aromatic Mediterranean plant, this asteraceae can grow to a height of 20–50 cm. The flowers are golden yellow and the foliage is silvery. The leaves are linear and very narrow. The flowers can be conserved for a long time and can be used to make dried flower bouquets. The name 'everlasting' comes from the exceptional longevity of the helichrysum flowers.

Botanical family:	Asteraceae
Part of the plant distilled:	Flowers
Taste:	Sour, sugary, herbaceous
Aroma:	Amber, spicy, reminding one of curry and hay

Principal components according to the gas chromatography of the essential oil: hyphenate ketones

History and mythology

Helichrysum comes from the Greek *helios* which means 'sun' and *chrysos* which means 'golden', and *italicum* is due to the region where the plant was described for the first time. Greek mythology associated helichrysum with Apollo, a god who used yellow flowers in his hair to remind the world of his immortality. Their medicinal qualities were ignored for a long time. The recognition of this plant in phytotherapy is in fact rather recent.

Experiences with everlasting hydrosol

Everlasting essential oil has been considered as the champion against haematoma for a long time. The hydrosol confirms this aspect. We can observe that, when ingested, it rapidly absorbs internal and external haematoma. Furthermore, it has a draining effect, and cures with this hydrosol help reduce cholesterol and glycaemic levels. It is excellent for treating cardiovascular troubles, such as haemorrhoids, varicose veins and rosacea. It accelerates the wound-healing process, so don't forget it for cases such as episiotomy, dental work, and after an operation.

Testimonial

'Each year, our school participates in an exhibition on natural medicine. While I was informing someone about our training, a wood panel fell off the metal structure and hit my nasal bone badly. My colleagues arrived on the scene with everlasting hydrosol that I swallowed pure (2 sips every 5 minutes, then I spaced out the sips). After a visit to a pharmacy for bandages, and a good night's sleep, I woke without haematoma or swelling on the face. My husband, after hearing the story, didn't believe it had happened, given that the effects of the accident were hardly visible.'

Energy and psycho-emotional properties

Everlasting links us to the eternity of the universe and at the same time to the strengths of the earth. It helps us remain rooted in reality and overcome psychological wounds. Blockages are not able to resist this master of energy purification. Everlasting absorbs 'blues' of the soul that prevent one from facing the present and future with serenity and confidence. The healing and purification of the past allows one to get to the bottom of things with more clarity and fewer mental projections. Treatment with this hydrosol is particularly useful for people who want to overcome a difficult childhood.

Properties and indications

* Absorbs internal and external haematoma: physical trauma, operations, episiotomy, dental work, broken bones, sprains

* Blood purifier, activates pancreatic and biliary vesicular functions, depurative: cholesterol, diabetes, obesity, metabolic problems, dermatosis, eczema, psoriasis

* Mucolytic, increases mucus fluidity: sinusitis, rhinitis, respiratory allergies

* Lymphatic and circulatory activator: venous stasis, varicose veins, haemorrhoids, heavy legs, rosacea, contusions, venous problems, oedema, phlebitis

Suggestions

* Tooth extraction and dental surgery: use as a mouthwash several times a day.

* Black eye or haematoma: use compresses with the hydrosol; let it work for 15–30 minutes. At the same time ingest the hydrosol (1–5 glasses of water a day with 1 tsp. of hydrosol in each glass).

* Oedema: use a compress by mixing the Everlasting hydrosol with salt water.

* Sprain or muscle tear: make a hydrosol and salt water compress.

* Take a cure after surgery to purify the physical and emotional shock.

* Spray the affected zone in case of fall or hit.

* Hypercholesterolemia: take the everlasting hydrosol and blend it with geranium, shiso, carrot, ledum, rosemary verbenon or juniper hydrosols.

* Capillary fragility: blend the everlasting hydrosol with cypress, sandalwood, vetiver, yarrow or angelica root hydrosols.

* Arthritis in the fingers: bathe hand with water mixed with sea salt, arnica oil and everlasting hydrosol.

Contraindication

You should not take more than 1 tbsp. a day for more than 40 days.

FRANKINCENSE – *Boswellia carterii*

Dissolve rigidity and develop your communications with all dimensions

Portrait of the plant

This tree, with a height of up to 6 metres, is characterised by bushy foliage and small white or pale pink flowers. Incisions are made on the trunk in order to collect a whitish resinous and aromatic substance. On hardening, this frankincense resin becomes like gum and takes on an orange/brown colour. It is then burned or distilled.

BOTANICAL FAMILY:	Burseraceae
PART OF THE PLANT DISTILLED:	Resin
TASTE:	Astringent, sour, soft
AROMA:	Musky, amber, powdery, smoky

Principal components according to the gas chromatography of the essential oil: monoterpenes

History and mythology

This is certainly the substance that has always been used in all cultures and religions during spiritual rituals. In the Hindu tradition, it is called *dhupa*, which can be translated as 'perception of the consciousness that is present throughout the universe and within every organism'. Ayurvedic doctors proclaim its merits and affirm that frankincense can dissolve anything that is rigid. Medication made with this gum or resin is called sallaki.

Experiences with frankincense hydrosol

Considered as the most important anti-inflammatory (articulations) in Ayurveda, and also as a lipid reducer, the hydrosol seems to confirm these properties. It is thus effective in cases of joint pain and rheumatism, but also to lower the cholesterol and triglyceride level. As a mouthwash, it calms gum inflammation.

As an auric or ambiance spray, it dissipates negative energy. One can instantly feel lighter and more confident.

> *Testimonial*
>
> 'One of my clients had many small and ungainly scars on his face after juvenile acne. I suggested spraying his face several times a day with a frankincense hydrosol combined with a serum rich in polyunsaturated fatty acids at night. I saw him 4 weeks later, and his look seemed more luminous and smooth. He told me that he felt that the hydrosol also had an "anti-stress" effect and he was better able to deal with his heavy workload.'

Energy and psycho-emotional properties

The hydrosol from this mystic plant helps us better accept fate, overcome the associated suffering, and find the strength necessary for a new start. Frankincense makes us more permeable to higher vibrations, lowers mental resistance and rigidity, and makes us more flexible and open. It broadens our conscience and increases the quality of prana (the life force that enters our body at birth). The path between the heart's chakra and the crown chakra becomes wider, and breathing becomes deeper and more regenerating. Spraying a room with frankincense hydrosol deeply purifies the air and creates the necessary space for meditation, communication and clarity of the mind.

Properties and indications

* Cerebral tonic, analgesic, ocular tonic: lack of clarity, dementia, conjunctivitis

* Anti-inflammatory, expectorant: bronchitis, chronic cough, throat inflammation, asthma, asthmatic bronchitis

* Cardiovascular tonic: tachycardia, pain in the heart region

* Carminative, bilirubin regulator: lack of appetite, bloating sensation, diarrhoea, colon inflammation, problems with taste

- Spasmolytic and analgesic: menstrual pain and spasms, premenstrual syndrome

- Antiseptic, diuretic, uterotonic, aphrodisiac: dysuria, urogenital inflammations, amenorrhoea, dysmenorrhoea, fibroids, sexual problems

- Cutaneous regenerator: asphyxiated or mature skin, wrinkles, eczema, dermatosis, rosacea

Suggestions

- For fibroids or haemorrhagic periods, undertake a 40-day cure by combining it with cistus hydrosol: 1 tbsp. of each hydrosol in 1 litre of water to drink during the day. Massage the lower stomach and lower back with the corresponding essential oils, blended with carrier oil. Use hydrosol compresses on the lower stomach.

- For rigidity, mental confusion, mistrust, inability to feel a connection with other people, undertake a 40-day cure (1 tbsp. in 1 litre of water to drink during the day). Use the hydrosol regularly as an auric spray.

- Spray a room with hydrosol to get rid of negative energy and purify ambient residues.

- Use the hydrosol as a cutaneous tonic or in a mask for mature and asphyxiated skin.

- Regularly use as a mouthwash and/or spray the gums to help with gum inflammation.

- For intestinal inflammation or diarrhoea, drink a cup of hot water with 1 tbsp. of hydrosol before meals.

Culinary advice

- Gives a smoky and sophisticated touch to smoothies and fruit juices.

Contraindications

None.

GERANIUM – *Pelargonium asperum*

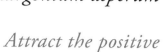

Attract the positive

Portrait of the plant

Originating from South Africa, today this plant is cultivated throughout the world. Its location strongly influences its biochemical composition. It can grow to 60 cm in height and has green cut leaves, jagged, with pink, red or white flowers.

BOTANICAL FAMILY:	Geraniaceae
PART OF THE PLANT DISTILLED:	Leaves
TASTE:	Soft, astringent, fresh
AROMA:	Flowery, rosy

Principal components according to the gas chromatography of the essential oil: monoterpenols, esters

History and mythology

The botanical name pelargonium comes from the Greek *pelargos*, which means 'crane', due to its elongated capsule in the form of a crane's beak. The geranium arrived in Europe at the end of the 17th century when the essence was used in perfumes for its fragrance. At the start of the 20th century, according to opera singers, it had the reputation of healing the voice and making it stronger.

Experiences with geranium hydrosol

Geranium has a pleasing aroma which charms the mind and makes it great as an auric or ambiance spray. It can be used for people who want to get out of difficult situations or create new perspectives. Its scent is much appreciated and often chosen for cutaneous and cosmetic creations. We can also spray the face during menopausal problems (hot flashes, depression).

Energy and psycho-emotional properties

A nervous system regulator, it fights stress and contributes to remaining focused. Geranium increases optimism and allows one to feel joy for no particular reason. It gets rid of blockages at the solar plexus level and as such helps one step back to look at judgements, projections and perceptions. It can reduce internal conflicts that prevent us from loving. As an auric spray, it creates an energy filter that transmits a feeling of protection and attracts positive situations.

Properties and indications

* Antispasmodic, anti-inflammatory, hepatic and pancreatic function activator, depurative: diabetes, stomach ulcers, intestinal inflammations

* Haemostatic, antiseptic, wound-healing: wounds, cuts, acne, rosacea, mycosis, eczema, impetigo, dermatosis

* Hormonal regulator: premenstrual syndrome, hormonal depression, amenorrhoea, cramps before periods

* Balances the cardiovascular system: hypertension, haemorrhoids, varicose veins, heavy legs

Suggestions

* Wounds, such as a child's scraped knee: spray the wound (soothes instantaneously).

* Depression, feeling like you're in a dead-end situation: leave a glass of water enriched with 1 tbsp. of hydrosol on the night-table, and drink on waking. Use the hydrosol during the day as an auric or an air spray.

* Bleeding haemorrhoids: sitz bath combining geranium hydrosol with other circulatory hydrosols (cistus, yarrow, cypress, sandalwood).

* Diabetes: undertake cures alternating with other depurative hydrosols.

* Cutaneous and nail mycosis: spray several times a day on the affected zone and also use the hydrosol internally.

* Hives, irritated skin and varied redness: spray several times a day on the affected zone, drink a glass of water enriched with 1 tsp. of hydrosol 3 times a day.

Culinary advice

* As a seasoning for carrots and red beets, spray at the end of cooking.

* Surprising and refined in cocktails and fruit juices.

* Matches perfectly with small red fruits: cranberries, raspberries, bilberries, strawberries, in sherbets, desserts and mousses.

Contraindications

None.

HYSSOP – *Hyssopus officinalis*

Align the chakras

Portrait of the plant

This is a perennial shrub that we can find throughout the Mediterranean basin. Its flowers are purple, white or red and grouped in spikes. Strongly aromatic, it attracts butterflies and bees. In general, the species is known for its resistance to drought and tolerance for limestone and sandy soils. It grows well in full sun and in warm climates.

BOTANICAL FAMILY:	Lamiaceae
PART OF THE PLANT DISTILLED:	Whole plant
TASTE:	Soft, astringent, fresh
AROMA:	Camphor, spicy

Principal components according to the gas chromatography of the essential oil: ketones

History and mythology

Hyssop is one of the medicinal plants known and used since antiquity. Its name comes from the Greek *hyssopus* or in Hebrew *esov* or *esob*, which means 'sacred herb'. The Bible advises (Psalm 51:7) 'Purify me with hyssop and I will be pure'. Some researchers believe that this refers to another plant from biblical times but nonetheless, phytotherapy confirms its purifying properties.

Experiences with hyssop hydrosol

Hyssop hydrosol confirms the mucolytic and expectorant virtues of the corresponding essential oil, evidently without contraindications. It is thus often used in mixes aimed at treating sinus infections, rhinitis, bronchitis, chronic coughs and respiratory allergies. This hydrosol can also be taken as needed to support work that requires a lot of concentration and focus.

Energy and psycho-emotional properties

Hyssop hydrosol helps clarity and lucidity by purifying Ajna, the third eye. It allows you to see things beyond the limits set by the mind. As an auric spray, it helps link the subtle bodies and purify the mind of all its previous beliefs. Thanks to this new clarity, it allows us to learn real lessons from experience. It purifies the aura of accumulated fear.

Properties and indications

* Astringent and antiseptic: flabby and asphyxiated skin, receding gums, tooth extraction or dental surgery, wounds, cuts, dermatosis

* Spasmolytic: respiratory spasm, asthma, muscular spasm, intestinal colic, acute abdominal pain

* Mucolytic and expectorant: cough, sinus infection, bronchitis, rhinitis

* Carminative, digestive, metabolic stimulant: aerophagia, intestinal gas, nausea, vomiting, slow metabolism

* Cardiac and nervous system tonic: convalescence, asthenic states, *kapha*-type depression

* Lymphatic and blood stimulant: venous stasis, oedema, cellulite

Suggestions

* As a hot compress on the forehead in case of sinus infection.

* A cup of hot water with 1 tsp. of hydrosol supports concentration and focus.

* Inhale in hot water in case of rhinitis or sinus infection.

Culinary advice

* Adds aroma to tomato-based dishes.

Contraindications

Hyssop essential oil, which contains 60–70 per cent monoterpenic ketones, is considered one of the more neurotoxic and abortive essences. This contraindication does not fully apply to the hydrosol. However, the use of this hydrosol should be avoided by pregnant women, epileptic people and young children.

JASMINE – *Jasminum officinalis*

Awaken your sensuality

Portrait of the plant

It's a climbing shrub with void foliage, semi-persistent, that flowers abundantly during the summer. It can reach 5 metres in height. Its very perfumed flowers are held by umbrella shaped treetops, both in the terminal and axial positions. It grows throughout Asia, in China, India, Vietnam and Thailand, in forests, hedges and along rivers. Jasmine is a shrub that is frequently cultivated in a mild and tropical climate. In the Mediterranean, it flowers from the end of June to September.

BOTANICAL FAMILY:	Oleaceae
PART OF THE PLANT DISTILLED:	Flowers
TASTE:	Sour, astringent, fresh
AROMA:	Sensual, flowery, a bit narcotic, intense

History and mythology

Jasmine is the flower whose virtues for lovers the Eastern poets extol. In Indian mythology, jasmine is associated with Kama, the god of eroticism (Kama = desire). With his bow, he shoots his jasmine arrows on people so that they fall in love. The flower is also used in temples as an offering, especially to Shiva. It seems that Cleopatra met Mark Antony on a boat with sails soaked in jasmine essence. Chinese and Ayurvedic medicine also proclaim the therapeutic merits of this plant, to which they attribute the following properties: relaxing, anti-depressant, aphrodisiac, as well as a metabolism stimulant, expectorant, antiseptic and anti-inflammatory. Some sources in Chinese medicine suggest using jasmine water to strengthen sperm.

Experiences with jasmine hydrosol

While this hydrosol has only recently appeared in the European market, it has long been used in hydrosol therapy. An excellent metabolic stimulator and depurative, it works ideally in a programme with other draining hydrosols. Its much-appreciated, sensual fragrance invites olfactory experimentation and it can be used as a cutaneous tonic.

Testimonial

'A 55-year-old friend who loved the perfume of this hydrosol often sprayed her body after a shower, added it to her tea and to her water during meals, sprayed sherbets, her bedroom before sleep, and so on. After a month of use, she had lost 2 kg (without following a particular diet) and in addition noted that her articular pain (knees, fingers) had disappeared. She also felt a new psychological lightness.'

Energy and psycho-emotional properties

Jasmine represents the message of luck that brings joy, love and abundance. Its intoxicating scent helps to detach the mind and invites it to let go. Having sattvic qualities, it increases the spiritual perception, helps to better feel the invisible and to develop love and compassion. Ayurveda associates it with lunar qualities: it freshens and calms mental agitation, stimulates optimism and transmits joy and happiness. It dilates the 2nd chakra, stimulates creativity and gives inspiration.

Properties and indications

* Analgesic, anti-inflammatory, antiseptic: rheumatism, gout, muscular pain, urogenital inflammation, migraines, styes, mouth ulcers

* Relaxing, anti-depressant, calming, nervous system tonic: pessimism, cartesian mind, cynical attitude, blandness, lack of integrity and loyalty, susceptibility, emotional fragility

* Astringent, diuretic, metabolic stimulant: hepatic and pancreatic insufficiency, bulimia, cravings for sugar, oedema

* Emmenagogue, aphrodisiac: amenorrhoea, dysmenorrhoea, fertility problems, impotence, frigidity

- Uterotonic: used during childbirth, it relaxes and helps with labour

- Expectorant, antiseptic: cough, bronchitis, fever

Suggestions

- During a diet, undertake a cure with jasmine hydrosol by adding 1–2 tbsp. in 1–2 litres of hot water to drink daily.

- After a stressful day, take a bath with 2 tbsp. of jasmine hydrosol. Also spray the bathroom before the bath.

- Spray the bedroom for more relaxing sleep or for couple's time.

- Spray the body after a day in the sun.

- Start to drink jasmine hydrosol 1 week before pregnancy due date for its uterotonic effect.

- Spray the affected zone in cases of mouth ulcers.

- Use compresses for styes.

Culinary advice

- Excellent to add aroma to tea, herbal teas, cocktails and fruit juices.

- Add to pastries, desserts, ice cream and sherbet.

- Very refined! A citrus salad flavoured with jasmine hydrosol…

Contraindications

None for olfactory and cutaneous uses. Avoid internally during pregnancy.

JUNIPER – *Juniperus communis*

Purify the body and mind

Portrait of the plant

This coniferous plant can grow up to 15 metres in height. Its trunk has grey rough bark; its leaves are small sharp needles, rigid, green, with a blueish white line. The fruit (juniper berries) are fleshy globe-shaped cones, first green, then black and waxy. It is at this moment that they are edible.

BOTANICAL FAMILY:	Coniferous
PART OF THE PLANT DISTILLED:	Shoots with needles and berries
TASTE:	Astringent, hot, sour
AROMA:	Spicy, woody, like gin

Principal components according to the gas chromatography of the essential oil: monoterpenes

History and mythology

Juniper wood was used in antiquity for purifying fumigation. It seems that Hippocrates fought the plague in Athens thanks to this fumigation. The Romans produced diuretic wines. In the Middle Ages, juniper was a universal remedy against demons and as a general tonic, as an antiseptic, diuretic, blood detoxifier and against rheumatism.

Experiences with juniper hydrosol

This is a powerful diuretic that acts quickly and stimulates kidney functions. It is also effective to reduce oedema and treat gout and rheumatism. It combines very well with other hydrosols that stimulate the metabolism, such as rosemary verbenon, jasmine or cypress. It also purifies at physical, psycho-emotional and energy levels.

Energy and psycho-emotional properties

Juniper helps one to get over psychological stagnation and restart one's life. It gives power, courage and willingness. A spiritual, mental and physical purifier, it helps find motivation and the necessary energy to evolve or accept change. It supports a pragmatic mind and the desire for action. It reduces *kapha* bioenergy and diminishes laziness and lethargy. It is very helpful for *kapha* people when they are going through demotivating and depressing periods.

Properties and indications

* Diuretic and anti-inflammatory: oedema, water retention, rheumatism, arthritis, gout, cellulite, sciatic nerve pain, lumbago, cystitis, prostatitis

* Stimulates blood and lymphatic circulation: lymphatic and venous stasis, hypotension, heavy legs and cellulite

* Hepatic, kidney and pancreatic stimulant, depurative: metabolic problems, obesity, difficult digestion, diabetes, hypothyroidism, hypercholesterolemia

* Antiseptic and depurative: acne, comedos

* Litholytic: renal lithiasis

* Anticatarrhale: rhinitis, cough (especially for *kapha* type)

Suggestions

* Obesity, difficult digestion, cellulite, oedema, water retention: undertake a 40-day cure (combined with other hydrosols, such as rosemary verbenon, cypress, everlasting, jasmine, sage), 1–2 tbsp. in 1 litre of hot water to

drink during the day (hot water is better at stimulating the digestive and metabolic process).

* Use in a foot bath to relieve heavy legs and cellulite.

* Cutaneous tonic: in a hydro-fomentation or mixed with a clay mask for oily skin, acne or comedones.

* Oedema, water retention: drink a cup of hot water with 1 tsp. of hydrosol 3–6 times a day.

* Feeling powerless, lack of motivation, fatigue: for 40 days, take 1 glass of hot water with 1 tsp. of juniper hydrosol on waking up. Inhale the essential oil of common or mountain juniper, with eyes closed, for 2 minutes.

* Use as an ambiance or auric spray to get rid of negative energy and purify the air.

Culinary advice

* As a seasoning for sauerkraut and broth.

* Creates an interesting aroma for sweet jams (strawberry, melon, peach).

* In depurative vegetable juices.

Contraindications

Important kidney problems. Pregnant women and children should avoid ingestion.

Kewra – *Pandanus odoratus*

Protect the heart

Portrait of the plant

The pandanaceaes are tropical plants that include more than 600 species found throughout Asia and Polynesia. The tree resembles a strange palm tree. Kewra flowers provide a delicious essential oil, which is rare and precious, and they make an exceptional hydrosol.

BOTANICAL FAMILY:	Pandanaceae
PART OF THE PLANT DISTILLED:	Flowers
TASTE:	Soft, astringent, fresh
AROMA:	Suave, piercing, amber, sensual

Principal components according to the gas chromatography of the essential oil: ethers

History and mythology

Kewra is used in Asia in cooking sweet dishes, but also in Ayurvedic medicine for its many virtues in the treatment of *sadhaka pitta*, the 'fire' aspect of bioenergy that manages and controls heart functions and also contributes to the clarity of the mind. Ayurvedic doctors regularly prescribe this plant, dedicated to Brahma (the Creator), for various problems: cardiac problems, rheumatism, headaches, accumulation of toxins in the liver, pancreas and intestines, but also for fever, diabetes, mental confusion, and the rajassic and tamassic attitudes of the mind. In Urdu, one of the languages used in northern India, it is called *ruh* which means 'refreshing for the soul'. Today, Ayurveda still uses this hydrosol to calm premature contractions during pregnancy and suggests that pregnant women drink this aromatic water regularly to protect the child.

Experiences with kewra hydrosol

The hydrosol confirms the properties attributed by Ayurvedic doctors. It harmonises cardiac functions, effectively fights metabolic and digestive problems, and is above all effective in cases of palpitations and arrhythmia.

Testimonial

'One of my patients suffered from menopausal problems, mood swings, and lack of emotional control. She had gained weight and her doctor had also diagnosed hypertension. I first suggested that she try "classic" hydrosols, such as clary sage, yarrow and also spikenard to balance her excess *pitta*. These hydrosols calmed her night sweats, her blood pressure was more stable and her emotions seemed more balanced. However, she said that she often felt different, isolated, alone… I suggested that she undertake a 40-day cure with kewra hydrosol. After about 10 days, she called me to say that she found the hydrosol fantastic and that, since using it, she felt that her heart was completely protected, as if certain worries and fears no longer mattered.'

Energy and psycho-emotional properties

People with healthy *sadhaka pitta* are mentally and emotionally balanced. They know how to recognise their role and are in agreement with themselves and with others. In effect, they find harmony between the body and mind, between the physical world and the spiritual dimension. Kewra acts deeply, and as such creates the necessary space to open one's heart and once again feel connections with others.

Properties and indications

* Balances emotions and nervous system: anger, attachment, mental confusion, neurasthenia, agitation, excessive emotions

* Analgesic, anti-inflammatory: arthritis, rheumatism

* Heart and nerve tonic: hypertension, palpitations, tightness in the heart, heart rhythm disorders

- Hepatic and pancreatic depurative: colic, diabetes, food cravings, headaches related to digestion, heartburn and gastric ulcers

- Cutaneous regenerator, antiseptic: hives, eczema, devitalisation of the skin, wounds

- Aphrodisiac: strengthens the functions of ovaries and testes (based on Ayurvedic medicine); libido disorders, frigidity, impotence, infertility, protects against miscarriages

- Antioxidant: immune deficiencies, cancer

- Very powerful antispasmodic: epilepsy, premature contractions, risky pregnancy

Suggestions

- If the heart has hardened as a result of disappointment, sorrow and so on, perform a 40-day cure with kewra hydrosol combined with the inhalation of the essential oils of rose, lemon verbena or champaca. Make compresses with kewra hydrosol on the heart.

- In the case of palpitations, arrhythmia, hypertension or metabolic problems, drink a cup of hot water with 1 tsp. of kewra hydrosol 3 times a day before meals. Use hot compresses on the solar plexus. Spray the face and heart.

- Spray the air in case of dense energy or if you are in a situation of conflict.

- Undertake a kewra hydrosol cure for 2–3 months in cases of immune deficiency.

- In pregnancy, drink a cup of hot water with 1 tsp. of kewra hydrosol 3 times a day and spray the stomach in case of premature contractions. Undertake a cure after the birth to recuperate faster.

Culinary advice

- Add to a vegetable or fish curry.

- It increases the antioxidant properties of green vegetable juice.

❈ Almond based desserts are delicious when flavoured with kewra hydrosol.

Contraindications

None.

Lavender – *Lavandula vera* or *angustifolia*

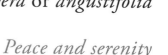

Peace and serenity

Portrait of the plant

This well-known lamiaceae is a perennial plant that takes the form of a shrub. It is made up of floral poles with a single spike and measures 30–60 cm in height. Growing at an altitude of 1000 metres, it originated in mountainous, limestone, dry and sunny regions of the Mediterranean. Today, it is cultivated throughout the world.

BOTANICAL FAMILY:	Lamiaceae
PART OF THE PLANT DISTILLED:	Floral peaks
TASTE:	Provencal, a bit sour, astringent
AROMA:	Flowery, honeyed, typical but nonetheless different from the essential oil

Principal components according to the gas chromatography of the essential oil: esters, monoterpenols

History and mythology

Lavender is a plant steeped in myth and legend; the Egyptians, Greeks and Romans proclaimed its merits. The name comes from the Latin *lavare* which means wash. The Hebrews used lavender for fumigation. Saint Hildegard of Bingen recommended it for liver problems. Pericles was convinced that it was a powerful tonic for nerves, and suggested its use in cases of mental illnesses. We can see that many cultures have considered lavender a 'general purifier'.

Experiences with lavender hydrosol

Along with orange blossom hydrosol, it is probably one of the most effective floral waters for sleeping. Lavender hydrosol calms *pitta*, razor burn, sunburns and dermatosis that 'burns'.

Energy and psycho-emotional properties

Lavender calms agitation, transforms rigidity, balances nervousness and purifies mental blockages. It relaxes a dense solar plexus when nervousness troubles digestion or creates fatigue, palpitations and hypertension. It brings harmony and balance during periods of agitation and calms stress. In this way, self-confidence is reinforced and we are able to face challenges in a more detached manner. It also supports therapies that aim to overcome educational patterns. Lavender awakens awareness in the crown chakra and battles arrogant, jaded and cynical behaviour.

Properties and indications

* Astringent, purifying, healing, refreshing and regenerating for the skin: acne, eczema, baby bottom erythema, prevents fleas, wounds, redness, sunburn, itchiness, razor burn

* Cardiac hypotensor and heartbeat regulator: hypertension, palpitations, arrhythmia

* Digestive, decreases the gastric acidity: gastric spasms (especially caused by nervousness), gastric acidity, bad breath, stomach ulcers

* Spasmolytic and analgesic: menstrual cramps, articulation and muscular pain

* Anti-stress: nervousness, agitation, fatigue

* Sedative: insomnia, difficulty falling asleep, jetlag

Suggestions

- If a baby doesn't sleep well, add 1–2 tbsp. of lavender hydrosol to the bathwater, and spray the bedroom.

- Use hot compresses on the stomach in cases of abdominal spasm.

- Spray the baby's bottom in cases of erythema.

- Spray the face after shaving to relieve sensitive skin, redness or razor burn.

- Spray the whole body after a day in the sun.

- Spray children's heads before going to school to prevent lice (mix 1–2 tbsp. of hydrosol with their shampoo).

- Use lavender ice cubes on insect bites to immediately soothe them.

- Spray pets to keep fleas away.

Culinary advice

- Gives a Provencal aroma to fruit salads, desserts, ice cream, crème brulée, and chocolate mousse.

- To impress your guests, make ice cubes with hydrosol and lavender blossoms for a great touch to cocktails.

- Add 1 tsp. of this hydrosol to 1 glass of apple juice to make a surprising and delicious drink.

Contraindications

None.

LEDUM – *Rhododendrum groenlandicum*

The fountain of youth

Portrait of the plant

Rhododendron groenlandicum (bog Labrador tea, formerly ledum groenlandicum or ledum latifolium) is a flowering shrub with white flowers and evergreen leaves. It is found in the tundra bogs and forests in northern Canada. It is a low shrub, growing to 50 cm and sometimes up to 2 metres. The leaves are wrinkled on top, densely hairy white to red-brown underneath, and have a leathery texture, curling at the edges. The tiny white flowers grow in hemispherical clusters and are very fragrant and sticky.

BOTANICAL FAMILY:	Ericaceae
PART OF THE PLANT DISTILLED:	Whole plant
TASTE:	Bitter, soft
AROMA:	Herbaceous, resin, recalls the smell of hay

Principal components according to the gas chromatography of the essential oil: monoterpenes, sesquiterpenes

History and mythology

Also called Labrador tea or Greenland ledum, this plant was and still is a 'cure-all' remedy for native North Americans. The aboriginals used it for respiratory and digestive disorders and for tuberculosis, but also as a spice for cooking and to flavour their beer.

Experiences with ledum hydrosol

Both the hydrosol and the essential oil are known for their exceptional ability to decongest and regenerate at the hepatic, kidney and pancreatic level.

Energy and psycho-emotional properties

Ledum acts as a true fountain of youth on mental, psychological and physical levels. It has a general purifying influence, and restores energy to mind and body. This detox awakens internal power and feeds the strength needed for action. It is much easier to persevere with decisions or to change direction. Fears, worries and destructive emotions dissipate. It calms tension in the solar plexus, allowing energy to circulate freely once again. A cold climate plant, its freshness calms symptoms of excess *pitta,* such as difficulty in controlling emotions, having a critical and tyrannical attitude, being judgemental, and having an inability to step back.

Properties and indications

- ❋ Depurative, calming: acne, sensitive and reactive skin, eczema, cutaneous allergies

- ❋ Detoxifying, hepatic, pancreatic and kidney regenerator, metabolic stimulant, decongestant: detox, hepatitis, pancreatic, hepatic and renal insufficiency, digestive problems, metabolic troubles, poor sleep caused by digestive problems

- ❋ Decongestant: prostatitis, nephritis, urinary inflammation

Suggestions

* Drink a cup of hot water with 1 tsp. of ledum hydrosol at night after a heavy meal for a better sleep.

* Undertake a 40-day cure at the end of summer (1 tbsp. per day in 1 litre of water) if you've accumulated too much *pitta*, meaning that you are continuously craving for food, you are irritable and anything can set you off...

* Undertake a 40-day cure to re-establish the body after an illness (chemotherapy, antibiotics, surgery).

* Spray the face after bathing in the case of acne; spray an eczema area or hives, use as a tonic and also internally in case of cutaneous allergies.

Contraindications

None.

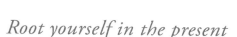

MARJORAM – *Origanum majorana*

Root yourself in the present

Portrait of the plant

This odorous perennial lamiaceae grows throughout the Mediterranean basin, and can reach 60 cm in height. Its stems have small white and purple flowers and oval leaves.

BOTANICAL FAMILY:	Lamiaceae
PART OF THE PLANT DISTILLED:	Whole plant
TASTE:	Bitter, soft, spicy
AROMA:	Hot, herbaceous, woody

Principal components according to the gas chromatography of the essential oil: monoterpenes, sesquiterpenes, monoterpenols

History and mythology

The botanical name *origanum majorana* comes from the Greek *oros ganos*, which means joy of the mountain. According to legend, Aphrodite, goddess of love, created this herb as a symbol of good fortune. The plant was also placed on tombs so that the dead were lucky in the afterlife and protected from evil spirits. Aristotle proclaimed its virtues and suggested it as an antidote to poisoning. The Greeks also massaged the scalp and the forehead with an oil enriched with marjoram to maintain a calm mind. In India, it is a sacred plant used to favour the resurgence of memories from past lives and to learn lessons from these experiences.

Experiences with marjoram hydrosol

Very calming, hypnotic and sedative, this hydrosol calms nervous spasm and agitation. It aids sleep and can also soothe articular, muscular, digestive or menstrual pain. Children who often have a sore stomach before exams or who are nervous and worried can be calmed with a hot compress of this hydrosol on the stomach.

Energy and psycho-emotional properties

Very balancing and harmonising, marjoram helps to traverse periods of turbulence and peaks of stress with calm and serenity. The hydrosol gets rid of fear, fights pessimism, destructive and negative attitudes and transmits the power necessary to take responsibility. Like its essential oil, marjoram hydrosol roots one in the present and as such supports a calm and lucid mind. This hydrosol dilates the heart chakra, calms tensions in the solar plexus, balances *vata* bioenergy and supports concentration.

Properties and indications

* Bactericidal, virucidal, fungicidal: colds and intestinal infections, cutaneous infections, urogenital infection

* Digestive: aerophagia, bloating, abdominal pain (above all due to nervousness)

* Calming, relaxing, hypnotic, vasodilator: insomnia, neurasthenia, psycho-emotional imbalance, hypertension, arrhythmia, tachycardia, palpitations, migraines

* Analgesic, decongestant, anti-inflammatory: muscular and articular pain, painful menstruations, back pain, dental infections and pain

* Nervous and balancing tonic at the level of thyroid functions: hyperthyroidism

Suggestions

* Hot compress on the abdomen in case of abdominal spasm.

- In case of hypertension, palpitations, arrhythmia: before each meal drink a cup of hot water with 1 tsp. of hydrosol and 3–5 times a day apply a drop of marjoram essential oil to the armpit, altering it with spikenard, lavender or ylang ylang.

- 1–3 tbsp. of marjoram hydrosol in bath water is relaxing and calming.

- Drink a cup of hot water with 1 tsp. of hydrosol before going to bed if tomorrow worries you.

- Use a hot compress and place it on the painful zone to sooth rheumatism.

Culinary advice

- Spray salads, vegetables and sauces.

- Mix with marinades, salad dressings and seaweed tartar.

- Add to fish sauces.

Contraindications

None.

MYRTLE – *Myrtus communis*

The joy of purity

Portrait of the plant

This shrub, which grows 2–3 metres in height, is found throughout the Mediterranean basin. The stems are covered with a reddish bark, and it has small white odorous flowers and small dark blue berries.

BOTANICAL FAMILY:	Myrtaceae
PART OF THE PLANT DISTILLED:	Leaves
TASTE:	Bitter, slight menthol taste
AROMA:	Green, reminiscent of eucalyptus but softer

Principal components according to the gas chromatography of the essential oil: oxides

History and mythology

The Greeks associated myrtle with Aphrodite, goddess of love and beauty. Even today, newlywed couples wear crowns of this plant as a sign of purity and beauty. An ancient Arab myth states that on leaving the Garden of Eden, Adam took a myrtle branch to remind him of his happiness there.

Experiences with myrtle hydrosol

As an expectorant, decongestant and mucolytic, this hydrosol is ideal for use as a nasal spray in cases of rhinitis, sinusitis and so on. People suffering from hay fever, eye inflammation, or red and itchy eyes can benefit from the calming and decongestant properties of myrtle. It can also be used as a cutaneous tonic in cases of acne, mycosis or rosacea.

Testimonial

'On a Saturday morning, I should make up a bride for her afternoon wedding ceremony. She came into my beauty spa with swollen eyes and red spots all over her face, she had tried a new cream the day before. She was overwhelmed by her emotions and in panic not being beautiful for the most in important day of her life! I sprayed her face with myrtle hydrosol, gave her a glass of water with 1 spoonful of this plant water to drink, than put a compress soaked in myrtle hydrosol on her face. After 15 minutes, the eyes were clearer and the spots disappeared. The bride had a healthy and fresh look again.'

Energy and psycho-emotional properties

The purifying and balancing virtues of this hydrosol help fight against addictions, and harmonise extreme emotions, nervousness and agitation. It links the heart chakra with that of the throat, thereby creating the necessary space to reinforce the physical and energy immune system. It dissolves obstinacy and makes people more open and flexible. It can be suggested to people suffering from addictions and self-destructive attitudes.

Properties and indications

* Expectorant, mucolytic, virucidal, antiseptic: rhinitis, sinusitis, bronchitis, cough, hay fever, gum inflammation

* Astringent, purifying, fungicidal: acne, dull and devitalised skin, rosacea, fungal infections

* Psycho-emotional balancer: addictions, self-destructive attitudes, obstinacy, agitation and scattered thoughts

* Decongestant, calming and purifying: sprains, oedema

* Antiseptic, eye decongestant and virucide: hay fever, eye inflammation, shingles of the eye

Suggestions

* Combine myrtle hydrosol with ravintsara hydrosol to treat shingles of the eye. Use compresses on the eyes, and regularly spray the eyes.

* To stop smoking, undertake a 40-day cure with 2 tbsp. of hydrosol in 1 litre of water to drink each day. At the same time, apply several drops of myrtle hydrosol on the thymus area. Smell hemlock fir, bergamot and myrtle essential oils to calm the need for a smoke.

* To treat fungal infections, use colon enemas or irrigations with myrtle hydrosol combined with tea tree, vetiver and geranium hydrosols.

* Use as a nasal spray to soothe upper respiratory tract congestion.

Culinary advice

* Add to herbal tea for respiratory problems.

Contraindications

None.

Orange blossom (or Neroli) – *Citrus aurantium*

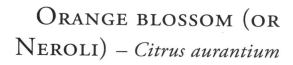

A glimpse of optimism

Portrait of the plant

This member of the rutaceae family grows 5–10 metres high and is also called bitter orange. It spread across India at the start of Christianity, and was introduced in the Mediterranean area during the Crusades. The Moors cultivated it intensively near Seville in Spain, which gave it the name Seville orange. The distilled leaves give the essential oil petitgrain bigarade and the essential oil of the blossom is often called neroli.

Botanical family:	Rutaceae
Part of the plant distilled:	Blossom
Taste:	Fruity, floral, sweet, astringent
Aroma:	Delicate, honeyed, sensual, fruity

Principal components according to the gas chromatography of the essential oil: monoterpenes, monoterpenols, esters

History and mythology

For many years orange blossoms have been renowned for their hydrosol and their essential oils across the Mediterranean basin. The hydrosol is considered as a sedative, prophylactic for gastrointestinal problems, weakness of the nervous system, gout, sore throats and insomnia. Orange blossom water is traditionally used in oriental pastries, desserts, liqueurs and cocktails, and so on.

Experiences with orange blossom hydrosol

Its calming and anxiolytic properties are very well known for insomnia, depression, stress, emotional shocks and so on. It calms agitated children and babies, and also animals. Spraying the animal before taking them to the vet allows them to remain calmer. It is also one of the best hydrosols for children who struggle with sleeping.

Energy and psycho-emotional properties

Orange blossom helps reconciliation with oneself and others. It purifies the body and mind and helps get rid of suffering and blockages. Like its essential oil, the hydrosol calms shock, depression and worry, and through its transmitted serenity it helps free one from so called 'dead-end situations'. It comforts sensitive and fragile people who find themselves in a crisis. It purifies the channel between the 2nd and the 5th chakra, and in so doing creates the necessary space for creative and calm communications.

Properties and indications

* Sedative: insomnia

* Anxiolytic, calming: depression, agitation, shock, stress, nervousness

* Comforting, calming: stopping smoking, alcohol use, anti-depressant drugs

* Emollient, cutaneous regeneration and softening: sensitive skin, baby skin, fragile skin, eczema, mature skin, dull skin

* Calming: anger, irritability

Suggestions

* Stopping smoking, use of alcohol and anti-depressant drugs: undertake a 40-day cure with 1 tbsp. of orange blossom hydrosol in 1 litre of water to drink during each day.

* Spray the baby's delicate skin.

- Insomnia: drink a glass of water or a cup of hot water with 1 tsp. of hydrosol before bed.

- Anger, agitation, frustration: take the same cure as for 'stopping smoking' and also smell neroli essential oil regularly.

- Delivering a baby: 1 week before term, the future mother can drink 1 litre of water with 1–2 tbsp. of orange blossom hydrosol on a daily basis. During labour, the mother can be sprayed with the hydrosol (face, belly, inner arms).

- Use as an auric spray to make one more receptive and open to others.

- For exams, drink 1 litre of water with 1–2 tbsp. of hydrosol the day of the exam. Use the hydrosol as auric spray before and during the exam. Massage wrists with some drops of neroli essential oil.

Culinary advice

- Much appreciated aroma in pastries, desserts, fruit salads and crepes.

- Matches perfectly with peaches, melon, apricots and figs.

- Gives a wonderful taste to fish and seafood sauces.

- Sharpens the taste of white cheese, lhassi and yogurts.

Contraindications

None.

Palmarosa – *Cymbopogon martinii*

Reassuring and soothing

Portrait of the plant

Palmarosa is a fragrant herb of Indian origin and comes from the family of cymbopogon, the same family as lemongrass, gingergrass and citronella. It grows in its wild form in dry soil on the banks of the Ganges and all the way to Afghanistan. It can grow to a height of 3 metres and has long and narrow leaves similar to citronella.

BOTANICAL FAMILY:	Grasses
PART OF THE PLANT DISTILLED:	Whole plant
TASTE:	Soft, fruity, suave
AROMA:	Flowery, rose, sensual

Principal components according to the gas chromatography of the essential oil: monoterpenoles

History and mythology

Ayurveda medicine recommends palmarosa to treat rheumatic pains, neuralgia, lumbago and sciatica, as well as fever and even hair loss. In oriental medicine, it is said to calm the 'fire'. Palmarosa refreshes, hydrates and reinforces yin energy. The natives of Caribbean islands love palmarosa both as a drink and as a skin tonic, and they are known for not suffering from acne.

Experiences with palmarosa hydrosol

It calms extreme emotions and guilt very effectively. Studies from the University of Gujarat on palmarosa hydrosol published in 2010 show that it has important protective effects for the central nervous system. Palmarosa can be considered as a neuro-protector. It is also effective for the treatment of epilepsy, headaches and anorexia.

Testimonial

'I've always had a feeling of guilt towards my father, and always felt that I disappointed him with my life choices. My therapist suggested that I undertake a 40-day cure with palmarosa hydrosol and massage my solar plexus and the kidney region with the same essential oil. I also used the hydrosol as an auric and air spray, especially before seeing my father. After 2 weeks of use, my mind was more serene, and I was able to talk to my father. It ended up being a deep discussion that resolved our issues and reinforced our reciprocal love, and since then I no longer feel guilty.'

Energy and psycho-emotional properties

Palmarosa hydrosol is subtle and flowery and has many psycho-emotional virtues. It deeply relaxes and removes psychological and mental torment linked to stress, guilt, attachment and perfectionism. As such, it is ideal for asthenic states, fatigue, and when nerves are frayed. It complements and reinforces the effects of rose, geranium, champaca and kewra hydrosols in helping us to let go of distressing issues. It reinforces *sadhaka pitta* functions.

Properties and indications

* Analgesic, relaxing, anxiolytic, lessens guilt: stress, neurasthenia, perfectionist mind, guilt, depression, frustration, anger, headaches, epilepsy, anorexia

* Bactericidal, virucidal, fungicidal, antiseptic, cutaneous tonic, astringent: dermatosis, eczema, acne, rosacea, reactive and sensitive skin, mycosis, wounds and sores

- Anti-inflammatory at the pancreatic, spleen and liver levels: calms excessive need for sugar, balances food behaviour problems, suggested for craving, excessive appetite

- Uterotonic, emmenagogue: amenorrhoea and dysmenorrhoea, premenstrual syndrome, haemorrhagic periods, childbirth

- Cardiac tonic: heart rhythm disorders, cholesterol, heavy and tired legs, haemorrhoids and varicose veins

Suggestions

- Used as an air spray it creates an interesting atmosphere, conveys a sense of euphoria and joy and subtly perfumes the room.

- In cases of excess *pitta*, with feelings of guilt, perfectionist mind and excessive appetite or cravings: undertake a 40-day cure with 1–2 tbsp. of hydrosol in 1 litre of water to drink during the day.

- Spray the hydrosol on the solar plexus and heart areas to feel better about oneself. Regularly spray the mouth in periods of mental rigidity or perfectionism.

- Use as a tonic for reactive skin or to calm razor burn.

Culinary advice

- Original in salad dressings for beets and carrots.

- Sophisticated in fruit cocktails and smoothies.

- Flowery and refined for muffins, fruit pies and mousses.

- Surprising in ice cream and sherbets.

- Softening in green tea.

Contraindications

The essential oil is considered as uterotonic, and until research says otherwise, it is better to avoid this hydrosol during pregnancy.

Peppermint – *Mentha piperita*

Invigorating and refreshing

Portrait of the plant

Peppermint is a perennial and hybrid plant. Its pale pink and slightly purplish flowers are formed in spikes. Its stem is reddish-purple. Today it is cultivated throughout the world.

BOTANICAL FAMILY:	Lamiaceae
PART OF THE PLANT DISTILLED:	Whole plant
TASTE:	Fresh, menthol
AROMA:	Menthol, fresh, herbaceous, spicy

Principal components according to the gas chromatography of the essential oil: monoterpenols

History and mythology

Legend states that mint came from Mentha, daughter of Cocytus, who fell in love with Pluto. Pluto's wife became jealous and crushed her with her foot. To save her, Pluto was only able to transform her into an odorous plant. Another legend states that mint grew in Venus's garden. In antiquity, they made crowns called Venus's Tiara. Mint is one of the medicinal plants most used by our ancestors.

Experiences with peppermint hydrosol

Peppermint is very popular in hydrosol therapy for its fresh taste, its stimulating and refreshing virtues and its spicy perfume.

Testimonies

'Children suffering from chicken pox are soothed if you spray the hydrosol on the pox. Excellent for calming explosive tempers and for fresher breath… A hydrosol that is excellent both therapeutically and for its taste.'

'One summer day, a corpulent patient had an appointment for a massage and she arrived covered in sweat, and was quite embarrassed by the situation. I gave her a glass of water with peppermint hydrosol, her sweating subsided, and then she was able to take full advantage of her treatment.'

Energy and psycho-emotional properties

Peppermint hydrosol develops clarity and freshness of mind and dispels confusion. It is effective for a wide variety of problems, including calming mental chattering and dissolving numerous fears. This hydrosol is not only an excellent digestive on a physical level but also symbolically. It helps 'deal with the past' to bring on new thoughts and concepts. Peppermint hydrosol calms explosive tempers, balances irritability and transmits clarity.

Properties and indications

* Astringent, refreshing, stimulating for microcirculation, antiviral: rosacea, inflamed acne, razor burn, weak microcirculation of the skin and dull complexion, itching, hives

* Lymphatic and venous stimulant: varicose veins, heavy legs

* Refreshing: excessive sweating, hot flashes

* Pancreatic stimulant: difficult digestion, metabolic disorders, difficulty to concentrate, lack of motivation, nausea, lack of appetite, motion sickness

* Antiviral, analgesic, calms itching: shingles, herpes, chicken pox, insect bites, migraines, sprains

Suggestions

* Use a cold compress with peppermint hydrosol on the forehead in case of migraines; spray the forehead and temples several times a day.

* Spray the whole body in cases of sunburn or hot flashes.

* Spray the forearms with the hydrosol to provide immediate refreshment on a hot day.

- Spray the affected zone in case of shingles, herpes or chicken pox; also drink 2–3 tbsp. diluted in water.

- Spray feet and legs after a walk or a night on the town; during long car trips, spraying the face from time to time with this hydrosol is invigorating.

- Add peppermint hydrosol to drinking water during the summer to keep *pitta* balanced.

Culinary advice

- Makes ice cubes for summer drinks.

- Gives a fresh taste to fruit salads and chocolate desserts.

- Spray on a lemon sherbet.

- Add 1 tsp. of hydrosol to green or black tea to give it a minty taste.

- Excellent for blending many drinks.

Contraindications

None.

SCOTS PINE – *Pinus sylvestris*

The taste of the forest

Portrait of the plant

The Scots pine is found in most of temperate and northern Europe, and spreads to eastern Siberia. It is a long, thin coniferous tree with a bare trunk and can live for 150–200 years. It reaches a height of up to 25 metres, and its needles can be 4–7 cm long.

BOTANICAL FAMILY:	Coniferous
PART OF THE PLANT DISTILLED:	Needles
TASTE:	Soft, fresh
AROMA:	Green, fresh, woody

Principal components according to the gas chromatography of the essential oil: monoterpenes

History and mythology

In eastern Europe, the pine is considered a protective tree against black magic and witchcraft. In Greece, the pine is called *pitys*. In mythology, Pitys was a nymph chased by Pan. She was transformed by the gods to escape the satyr. The Greeks associate the pine with Dionysus, and the Romans with Bacchus, the god of wine and pleasure, but also of abundance and fertility. The Celts associated the pine with the sun that lightened the obscurity of winter, and they honoured it during the winter solstice as they believed that the pines encouraged the sun to come back. Hippocrates suggested using it to treat pulmonary problems. According to Ayurveda, pine hydrosol reduces *vata* and *kapha* and stimulates Agni, the digestive fire.

Experiences with pine hydrosol

Drinking this hydrosol and/or spraying the body is reinvigorating, revitalising and regenerating for body and mind. In periods of lethargy, fatigue and also in cases of respiratory infection, it helps us find strength. It is often suggested for smokers or those who want to stop smoking in order to strengthen and detoxify the respiratory system.

Energy and psycho-emotional properties

The pine often grows on rocks, onto which it courageously hangs with its strong roots, which draw out the maximum nourishment. Its hydrosol transmits this strength, dilating the heart chakra, helping us to overcome existential crises and find the intuition to conserve resources. It purifies the heart of residues of sadness, mourning and sorrow, and lets us feel once again the connection with others, developing compassion and empathy. It fights susceptibility and helps relativise criticisms.

Properties and indications

* Depurative, draining, diuretic: cellulite, venous and lymphatic stasis, oedema, metabolic problems

* Mucolytic, expectorant, respiratory tonic: respiratory tract congestion, cough, bronchitis, smoker's cough, asthma, pharyngitis, sinusitis, pneumonia

* Analgesic, anti-inflammatory, decongestant: rheumatism, arthrosis, prostatitis, cystitis, general muscular and articular pain, sciatic nerve, sprains, blows

* General tonic: immune deficiency, asthenic states, hypotension, chronic fatigue, nervous exhaustion, depression, convalescence

* Antiseptic and fungicidal: dermatosis, acne, dull complexion and weak microcirculation of the skin, eczema, oily skin, mycosis

* Depurative, metabolic and gallbladder stimulant: hypothyroidism, obesity, constipation, food intolerance, gallstones

* Adrenal stimulant: sexual asthenia, fatigue

Suggestions

* In case of respiratory infection: combine with other suitable hydrosols, inhale, drink hot water enriched with hydrosols, gargle, and regularly spray

the throat. Add to a child's bath water. Use hot compresses enriched with hydrosol on the thorax.

* Use hot compresses on a painful zone such as a sprain, on painful articulations, on muscles after sports; also use in bath water.

* In cases of exhaustion and fatigue, undertake a 40-day cure with 1 tbsp. of pine hydrosol in 1 litre of water per day. At the same time, smell the essential oil.

* Smokers who want to stop can combine myrtle hydrosol with Scots pine hydrosol.

* Smokers with cellulite can combine cypress, myrtle, helichrysum, juniper and Scots pine hydrosols.

Culinary advice

* Gives a fresh and invigorating taste to homemade syrups.

* Add in infusions and green tea as a metabolic stimulant.

* Gives a sophisticated taste to peach or melon sherbet.

Contraindications

Can be a slight laxative; avoid using during pregnancy.

Ravintsara – *Cinnamomum camphora*

Look beyond

Portrait of the plant

The cinnamomum camphora, or ravintsara, from Madagascar is a large evergreen tree that grows up to 20–30 metres tall. The bright green leaves have a glossy and waxy appearance and give off a strong odour of camphor when rubbed. In spring, small white flowers appear. The fruits are small, black and look like little berries.

Botanical family:	Lauraceae
Part of the plant distilled:	Leaves
Taste:	Bitter, slight menthol
Aroma:	Green, fresh, camphor recalling eucalyptus

Principal components according to the gas chromatography of the essential oil: oxides

History and mythology

Originally from Madagascar, its name comes from the Malagasy *ravina*, which signifies leaf, and *tsara*, which means good. The Malagasies sell many plant species that have medicinal virtues for which they use this name, and that is why aromatherapy pioneers, such as Pierre Franchomme, originally gave it an erroneous botanical name (ravintsara aromatic). The hydrosol described below is in fact a camphor tree, for which we kept the original name to avoid the confusion that surrounds this hydrosol and its essential oil. Ravintsara essential oil has for a long time been one of the bestselling antivirals.

Experiences with ravintsara hydrosol

The hydrosol perfectly completes the antiviral virtues attributed to the essential oil. Although it has only recently become available, I have been able to note its effectiveness when sprayed on chicken pox with children, and also in case of herpes.

Energy and psycho-emotional properties

Its perfume activates the third eye, Ajna, and opens the door to the subconscious. It awakens lost memories, ancestral memories, helps one become conscious of ancient resources, our mental mechanisms, our attitudes and our beliefs. It soothes pain and allows for deep introspection.

Properties and indications

* Virucidal, mucolytic, expectorant, antiseptic: all viral infections – colds, respiratory tract infections, bronchitis, flu, nasopharyngitis, whooping cough, hepatitis, viral enteritis, shingles, herpes, chicken pox, mononucleosis

* Analgesic, supports flexibility of the joints: rheumatism, arthrosis, muscular and articular pain

* Sedative, balances mental and psycho-emotional disorders, relaxing, neurotonic: insomnia, depression, worry, agitation

* Immune booster: immune deficiency, chronic respiratory infections

Suggestions

* Herpes, shingles and chicken pox: spray the affected zone. Add 1–2 tbsp. (1–2 tsp. for children) to 1 litre of water to drink during the day. Can also be combined with peppermint hydrosol for adults.

* Shingles of the eye: spray the eyes, use compresses and drink 1–2 tbsp. in water during the day.

- Insomnia, worry, agitation: spray the solar plexus with hydrosol; before bed drink a cup of hot water with 1 tsp. of ravintsara hydrosol. Regularly inhale the corresponding essential oil.

- To prevent colds, add 3 tbsp. of hydrosol for an adult or 1 tbsp. for a child to bath water. Drink a cup of hot water with 1 tbsp. of hydrosol once a day.

Contraindications

None.

ROSE – *Rosa damascena*

Awaken the heart

Portrait of the plant

The Damascus rose is a hybrid mix of *rosa gallica* and *rosa moschata*. It is above all noted for the intense smell of its petals. It can grow in the wild in cool climates, but is also cultivated in the south. The main area of production today is in Bulgaria. The Damascus rose can grow up to 2 metres in height. The perfume is particularly intense before sunrise, and the best quality for both hydrosol and essential oil comes from fresh petals.

BOTANICAL FAMILY:	Rosaceae
PART OF THE PLANT DISTILLED:	Petals
TASTE:	Soft, fresh, velvety
AROMA:	Flowery, sensual, soft

Principal components according to the gas chromatography of the essential oil: monoterpenols, esters

History and mythology

Rose, the queen of flowers has symbolised love since antiquity and has always provided endless fascination. In most civilisations, the rose symbolises love, purity and passion. The Christian Holy Mother is often represented with a rose in her hand. Cleopatra supposedly covered the floor in her bedroom with a carpet of roses in order to encourage the Emperor Mark Anthony to fall for her charms. In Egypt, it is considered a universal remedy. In Greek mythology, it is said that the original colour of the rose was white and that it was the blood of Eros or Aphrodite, after a foot wound, that gave its red colour and divine perfume.

Experiences with rose hydrosol

We can observe that taking this hydrosol considerably calms explosive tempers. Spraying it in a child's room when they are having a tantrum, in a conference room where there is conflict and when each person refuses to budge, can be miraculous.

Additionally, it is an excellent remedy against the effects of an excess of *pitta*, from inflamed eyes to cutaneous eruptions, from excess appetite to overflowing emotions.

Testimonials

'I have a tough job, where I have to manage 1000 things at the same time, and where it is important to be vigilant and balanced. When I am challenged by someone and I feel about to explode, I drink a glass of water with 1 tsp. of rose hydrosol and I spray it around me, on my face, neck and around the heart area. I immediately feel refreshed, serene and more receptive.'

'I am dominated by *pitta* bioenergy. I am normally in a very bad mood before my period, and have long suffered from haemorrhagic periods. Doctors only suggested I do one thing: contraceptive pills that I can't really tolerate. Hydrosol therapy did wonders in less than a month of use. I mixed equal parts of cistus, rose and clary sage hydrosols and drank 1 litre of water with 1 tbsp. of this mix a day. For the first time in a long time, my period was "normal" and I felt serene and at peace before and after menstruation.'

Energy and psycho-emotional properties

Like its essential oil, rose hydrosol dilates the heart chakra and makes one more open and receptive. It balances emotions and dissolves blockages at the subtle body level. It calms excess fire in the body, and is excellent when one is struggling with love, mourning, anger, irritation and aggressiveness. Rose hydrosol also dissolves rigidity at the solar plexus and as such fights against an egotistical attitude. It draws one towards the experience of love, and allows one to feel more connected to others.

Properties and indications

* Astringent, purifying, tonifying, refreshing, anti-wrinkle, anti-inflammatory, analgesic: dull skin, cutaneous eruptions, nappy rash, older skin, allergic cutaneous reactions, wounds, sunburn, hives, itching, thrush

- Anti-inflammatory for the eyes: red and inflamed eyes, conjunctivitis

- Euphoria-inducing, anxiolytic, calming, neurotonic, anti-*pitta*: excessive appetite, hyperemotivity, bad breath, heartburn, excessive need for sugar, premenstrual syndrome, anger, frustration, fears, agitation, cynicism

- Aphrodisiac: sexual problems, lack of openness, inability to feel love and pleasure

- Regulator for respiratory, antiseptic: bronchitis, especially psychosomatic-based

Suggestions

- For a 40-day cure, drink 1 tbsp. in 1 litre of water per day to rebalance emotions, develop serenity and harmonise the mind.

- Drink a cup of hot water with 1 tsp. of hydrosol before meals to alleviate excessive appetite.

- During premenstrual syndrome, stomach cramps or bad mood before periods, use rose hydrosol as an ambiance spray. Drink 1 litre of water with 1 tbsp. of hydrosol per day starting 10 days before the start of your period.

- Spray yourself with hydrosol when feeling frustration and irritation.

- Add 2–3 tbsp. of hydrosol to bath water to feel refreshed after a tiring day.

- Spray the affected zone several times a day in cases of nappy rash, hives and cutaneous eruptions.

- Use vaginal douches for vaginal itching or burning, and spray the genitals several times a day: mix $1/3$ hydrosol with $2/3$ water.

- Regularly spray your eyes during continuous work in front of the computer.

Culinary advice

- Gives a sophisticated taste to raspberry, strawberry or blueberry desserts.

- Adds flavour to rice pudding.

- Delicious in smoothies and fruit juices.
- Adds imagination for sherbets, ice creams and white cheeses.

Contraindications

None.

ROSEMARY VERBENON – *Rosmarinus officinalis, ct. verbenoniferum*

Awaken the vital spirit

Portrait of the plant

Rosemary is a shrub that grows wild throughout the Mediterranean basin, in particular in France, in arid and rocky garrigues and in limestone soil. It can be cultivated in gardens. It has numerous phytotherapeutic virtues, and is also used for cooking. It is considered to be a honey-producing plant (rosemary honey is renowned), as well as an ingredient used in the manufacture of perfume.

BOTANICAL FAMILY:	Lamiaceae
PART OF THE PLANT DISTILLED:	Whole plant
TASTE:	Strong odour of fresh grass
AROMA:	Fresh, herbaceous, camphor, aromatic

Principal components according to the gas chromatography of the essential oil: monoterpenes, ketones

History and mythology

In antiquity, the Egyptians, Greeks and Romans often used rosemary during holidays and spiritual ceremonies. Rosemary was often the symbol for ancestral memory, which is why it was used during marriages in order to remember significant events or during burials in order to remember those who died. Greek students wore rosemary garlands to strengthen their memory. In the Middle Ages, this plant was used in medicine and in cases of hepatitis or when memory was weak, as well as for many other illnesses. The Latin term *rosmarinus* means 'dew of the ocean'.

Experiences with rosemary verbenon hydrosol

Rosemary verbenon hydrosol is an excellent remedy to stimulate the digestive fire and the function of liver, pancreas and kidneys. It is also excellent for stimulating the metabolic system and therefore is often used in depurative cures. We can also observe that people suffering from chronic rhinitis linked with food intolerance feel revitalised and in better shape after a cure with this hydrosol. Internal cures are often effective for people suffering from acne. It is one of the most effective hydrosols for reducing *kapha*.

Testimonials

'I used to suffer from fatigue in the spring, leaving me lethargic and worn out. Since I undertook a 40-day cure with rosemary verbenon hydrosol at the start of the spring, my vitality remains intact.'

'When I was taking personal development classes, I tended to fall asleep during meditation. So, I decided to drink rosemary verbenon hydrosol during the class. Since then, I hear each word with extraordinary clarity and have the feeling that it is clearly stored in my brain.'

'Two years ago, my mother hurt her foot and the wound became seriously infected. The doctor strongly urged her to take antibiotics, and spoke about the serious consequences if she didn't. However, my mother refused these antibiotics, and started to rinse the wound several times a day with rosemary verbenon hydrosol, then applied antibacterial, healing and anti-inflammatory essential oils. Rosemary verbenon hydrosol was key for the cleaning and drying of the wound.'

Energy and psycho-emotional properties

Rosemary is a very resistant plant that survives in arid regions and quickly grows back after fires. It activates the transforming fire inside us, and removes lethargy. It purifies the body and mind, reinforces memory, and supports concentration. It is an excellent tonic and very beneficial when we feel exhausted. It can be used in case of stagnation, when there is a blockage in the healing process. In this case, it triggers a new momentum and creates the vital strength necessary to continue.

Properties and indications

- Astringent, purifying, tonifying, refreshing: acne, dull and flabby skin, cellulite, combination skin

- Digestive, regenerating for the liver, gallbladder, pancreas and kidneys: weight gain, metabolic and premenopausal problems, water retention, lack of power, weight gain before period, prostatitis

- Cardiovascular stimulant: hypertension

- Mucolytic and expectorant: rhinitis (especially linked to allergies or food intolerance), chronic cough

- Nervous or mental tonic: poor memory, poor concentration, lack of clarity, pessimistic attitude, lack of motivation, difficulty in learning foreign languages, fear of facing a conflictual situation with others

Suggestions

- For a depurative cure or to activate the metabolism in pre-menopause, for 40 days, take 1 tbsp. of hydrosol in 1 litre of hot water.

- In the case of chronic rhinitis, drink 1 tsp. of hydrosol in a cup of hot water after meals twice a day. Place 1 drop in each nostril in the morning.

- For upper respiratory tract congestion (sinusitis), place a hot compress on the forehead and chest.

- For acne, drink a cup of hot water with 1 tsp. of hydrosol 1–2 times a day, use clay masks 1–2 times a week, and use the hydrosol as a tonic.

- Spray the face and forearms when having difficulty waking up.

- Take a bath with sea salt and 2–4 tbsp. of hydrosol after a tough day.

- During intensive study periods or exams, regularly spray the face and forearms; take baths with rosemary verbenon hydrosol.

- It is recommended to undertake a 40-day cure with rosemary verbenon hydrosol. At the start of the spring (the *kapha* period according to Ayurveda and the season where the liver must be stimulated according to Chinese medicine), add 1 tbsp. in 1 litre of water to drink on a daily basis.

❋ For late periods, apply hot compresses on the stomach and drink a cup of hot water with 1 tbsp. of rosemary hydrosol 1–3 times a day.

Culinary advice

❋ Add at the end of cooking for ratatouilles, carrots and celery.

❋ Use as a condiment for Mediterranean meals and tomato sauces.

❋ Gives a delicious taste to boiled potatoes.

❋ Surprising: pears in wine with a drop of rosemary verbenon hydrosol.

❋ Stimulant: 1 tsp. of rosemary verbenon hydrosol in a glass of pear juice.

Contraindications

Pregnancy and children under 3.

SAGE – *Salvia officinalis*

Awaken your internal power

Portrait of the plant

Sage officinalis is a bush of the lamiaceae family, often cultivated in gardens for cooking. Like most ketonic plants, its foliage is velvety and silvery, its flowers purple. Common in southern regions of Europe, it is rare to find it in the wild. It is a perennial and can grow to 1 metre in height.

BOTANICAL FAMILY:	Lamiaceae
PART OF THE PLANT DISTILLED:	Whole plant
TASTE:	Bitter, astringent
AROMA:	Terpene, camphor, herbaceous, resinous

Principal components according to the gas chromatography of the essential oil: ketones, oxides

History and mythology

The healing reputation of sage has been known since ancient times. In Latin *salvia* means 'heal' or 'save'. An ancient Latin text declares: 'Why a man who has sage in his garden has to die?' For the Romans, it was simply the *herba sacra*, the sacred herb.

Experiences with sage hydrosol

Used above all for menopausal problems, sage hydrosol is also very effective for excessive sweating.

Testimonial

'I suffered from hot flashes and water retention at the start of my menopause. A blend of equal parts of sage and vitex hydrosols made the hot flashes disappear quickly, and I was less bulimic. I had lost 2 kg within 3 weeks after the first use.'

Energy and psycho-emotional properties

Sage opens Ajna, the third eye or 6th chakra, supports letting go, heals wounds from the past, cleanses and refreshes our environment and creates a new life space. This process helps us to accept change and opens us up to meet new people and new situations. People who normally consider changes and separations as a loss can feel that in reality they are often more like new starts. Balancing *pitta* and *kapha*, sage calms bulimia and emotional overflows. It is also effective for purifying the air when the energy is dense and heavy. It helps us to remain focused and concentrated with an open mind free from stubbornness.

Properties and indications

* Oestrogen-like, emotionally harmonising, slight diuretic and lymphatic stimulant: menopausal problems, amenorrhoea, dysmenorrhoea, hot flashes, bloated stomach and cramps during periods, excessive need for sugar before menstruation, water retention during menstruation

* Analgesic, antibacterial, healing, fungicidal and anti-inflammatory: mouth ulcers, gum inflammation, wounds, cutaneous infections, mycosis

* Mucolytic: cough, rhinitis, bronchitis

* Calms the digestive fire, anti-*pitta*: cravings, excessive appetite before and during periods, excessive appetite at the start of menopause

* Antiperspirant, anti-hypersalivation: excessive sweating, hypersalivation

* Stimulates the lymphatic and venous system: lymphatic stasis, swollen ganglions, cellulite

* Astringent, protects against free radicals: oily skin, rosacea, mature skin

* Balances the functions of liver, pancreas, spleen and kidneys, digestive and diuretic, depurative: metabolic problems, difficult digestion, bulimia, obesity, water retention (caused by hormonal problems), hepatic and pancreatic insufficiency, cholesterol

* Mucolytic: colds, sinusitis, chronic cough

Suggestions

- In case of periodontitis, bleeding gums, mouth ulcers or gingivitis, use sage officinalis hydrosol as a mouthwash.

- During hot flashes and menopausal troubles, undertake a 40-day cure with this hydrosol: 1 tbsp. in 1 litre of water to drink during each day.

- In combination with cedar hydrosol, to favour hair growth and revitalise the scalp, rub the scalp with a mix of equal parts or add to shampoo.

- In case of excessive sweating, add 2 tbsp. of hydrosol to bath water or spray the feet and armpits after the shower. Drink a glass of water with 1 tsp. of the hydrosol.

- Apply hot compresses to the face before using a regenerating mask.

- Use with detox cures, as this works well.

Culinary advice

Gives a slightly sour and typical taste to sauces and marinades.

Contraindications

Pregnancy, children, mastosis or hormone-dependent cancer.

SANDALWOOD – *Santalum album*

Remain open

Portrait of the plant

Sandalwood trees grow in India, Nepal, Australia, New Caledonia and Hawaii. This evergreen tree grows 4–9 metres and can live to 100 years of age. The bark is reddish or dark brown and smooth in young trees;. leaves are thin, opposite and ovate to lanceolate in shape. The International Union for the Conservation of Nature (IUCN) recognised santalum album as a 'vulnerable' species. Due to its scarcity, sandalwood is not allowed to be cut or harvested by individuals and the Indian government is strictly controlling the cultivation of this majestic tree.

BOTANICAL FAMILY:	Santalaceae
PART OF THE PLANT DISTILLED:	Wood
TASTE:	Aromatic, woody, a bit sour, soft
AROMA:	Hot, woody, smoky

Principal components according to the gas chromatography of the essential oil: sesquiterpenols

History and mythology

Sandalwood, cultivated in India over the past 4000 years, is dedicated to the deity Vishnu. Traditionally associated with Buddhist and Hindu rituals, it fosters the discovery of the inner self, soothing the human ego and transforming it into spiritual wisdom. Its history is linked to that of the cultural, medicinal and spiritual life in Asia. Ayurveda and Chinese medicine proclaim its multiple therapeutic virtues.

Experiences with sandalwood hydrosol

Sandalwood hydrosol calms anger and irritability. It is a vital elixir for the circulatory system, arrhythmia, hypertension, haemorrhoids and varicose veins. It also helps with back pain, especially in the lumbar area but also at the cervical level. It is highly beneficial during a heatwave if one suffers from heavy and painful legs.

Drinking water enriched with this hydrosol during the summer helps us feel physically and psychologically lighter in the heat. A powerful decongestant and anti-inflammatory, it often works well for chronic urinary inflammation. It should also be used in case of a chronic nervous cough.

Testimonials

'A sitz bath with this hydrosol when I suffer from urinary infection or inflammation calms the burning sensation.'

'My 45-year-old patient suffered from terrible pain in her hips and lower back for several months. She went to see a rheumatologist who diagnosed ankylosing spondylitis. The first week, she took anti-inflammatory drugs, but she quickly felt intense pain in the stomach and was no longer able to sleep. I suggested that she take sandalwood and everlasting hydrosol (in total 2 tbsp. per day in her water) with a preparation of anti-inflammatory essential oils to apply locally. There was a clear improvement in the symptoms and she was quickly able to sleep again. She was able to reduce the anti-inflammatory drugs to the point of stopping them, and continued with the hydrosol as necessary.'

Energy and psycho-emotional properties

Sandalwood is considered to be a sacred plant in Asia and its hydrosol confirms its spiritual virtues. In an auric spray, it purifies the body and subtle channels (meridians, srotas). In Ayurveda, it is given a sattvic quality, meaning that it brings clarity and serenity. Cures with this refined hydrosol create the necessary space to get rid of old mental habits that prevent progress. It calms the ego and helps one to be at peace with oneself and with others. Vision becomes clearer, we are able to take a step back, and our mental state becomes more flexible and open.

Properties and indications

* Neurotonic and calming: dissolves nervous tension, scattered thoughts and mental agitation. It also calms nervous-based migraines

* Antiseptic and immuno-stimulant: chronic nervous cough

* Cardiac tonic: the majority of cardiac weaknesses, such as varicose veins, haemorrhoids, hypertension, arrhythmia, coronary inflammation and cellulite

* Digestive and anti-inflammatory: corrects taste and helps feel satiety, helps in cases of bulimia and gastric acidity, and calms pain linked to stomach ulcers

* Anti-inflammatory, analgesic, diuretic: urogenital inflammations, prostatitis, cystitis (also for prevention), rheumatism, arthritis

* Aphrodisiac: impotence, frigidity

* Astringent, anti-inflammatory and calming for the skin: rosacea, hives, dermatosis, acne

Suggestions

* During very hot weather, add sandalwood hydrosol to water (1 tbsp. for 1 litre).

* Spray sandalwood hydrosol in a room before meditating in order to clear the air.

* In cases of bulimia, and the inability to feel satiety, drink a glass of hot water enriched with 1 tsp. of sandalwood hydrosol before meals.

* At the end of cooking, adding 1 tbsp. to rice water protects against gastric acidity and is a great accompaniment to an exotic curry.

* With a chronic nervous cough, boil a piece of ginger (about the size of a finger) in 500 ml of water. Let the water cool to room temperature, then mix 300 ml of the concoction with 200 ml of sandalwood hydrosol and add 3 tbsp. of honey. Stir well and drink 1 small glass (about 15–20 ml) 3 times a day.

* For stomach ulcers, drinking 1 glass of hot water with 1 tsp. of sandalwood hydrosol calms the pain.

Culinary advice

* Use it in rice water at the end of cooking to generate a lovely woody taste.

* Gives a sophisticated taste to hot chocolate.

* A broth with sandalwood and coriander hydrosol served before the meal helps digest heavy meals and creates a feeling of satiety.

Contraindications

None.

Shiso – *Perilla frutescens*

Become flexible

Portrait of the plant

This lamiaceae, purple in colour, is native to East Asia and considered to be a medicinal plant in China, India, Japan, Korea, Thailand and Vietnam. In the 19th century, Asian immigrants brought the plant to the United States, where it was named 'beefsteak plant', as on the one hand, it helps store meat, and on the other, its large red leaves are reminiscent of a rare steak. Shiso is both a spice and a powerful medicinal plant, and it attracts a lot of butterflies. The whole plant is known for being rich in vitamins, bioflavonoids and minerals. Its essential oil provides a very rare aldehyde.

BOTANICAL FAMILY:	Lamiaceae
PART OF THE PLANT DISTILLED:	Whole plant
TASTE:	Soft, bitter, astringent
AROMA:	Spicy, woody, soft, amber, mysterious

Principal components according to the gas chromatography of the essential oil: perilla-aldehydes, monoterpenes, sesquiterpenes

History and mythology

In traditional Chinese and Japanese medicine, shiso is used as an anti-asthmatic, antibacterial, antidote for food poisoning, antipyretic, spasmolytic, anti-cough, digestive tonic, nervous system balancer, regenerator and expectorant. The chemical components of the essential oil confirm these properties, and recent studies have shown an effect against cancer. In certain Asian regions, notably in Japan, spiritual ceremonies are conducted before harvesting the plant as it is considered sacred, and divine, and sent by the Creator to save Man. The belief still exists that walking on the plant in a disrespectful way brings on illness and death. Taiwanese aboriginals plant shiso in their gardens to attract divine protection and to purify the surroundings. In the West, this plant can be called perilla, from its botanical name. Shiso is the Japanese name for the plant.

Experiences with shiso hydrosol

I discovered this hydrosol and its essential oil during a visit to Taiwan, where I was giving a class. My friend Yo June Wang, well-known author and teacher in Asia, proclaimed the merits of this plant and had even mentioned the research on the plant taking place at Taipei University. Its fragrance seduced me even before I was able to experiment with it. The essential oil and hydrosol were used very successfully as soon as they became available in Switzerland. Many testimonies highlight its exceptional anti-inflammatory virtues, and therapists successfully use it in cases of diabetes and cholesterol, and also to reinforce the immune system in cases of cancer.

Testimonial

'My doctor diagnosed elevated cholesterol and tryglizeride levels. I then drank a liter of water with 2 tablespoons of Shiso-hydrosol daily for 6 weeks. At the next check, my values were back to normal … But I also lost 2 kg without any changes in my eating habits.'

Energy and psycho-emotional properties

Shiso helps us to realise that the intellect cannot be smart until spiritual awareness awakens the higher octave of intelligence. Our mind becomes shaped by the collective consciousness and our experiences, and these create projections and limits. That is the reason why it is rare for us to fully exploit our potential and skills, and so the flame of life is always reduced. We thus become jaded, because we mistakenly think that we know everything and have answered all questions. The unique perfume of shiso is spicy, woody, bitter and soft at the same time. It is amber and mysterious and transmits a feeling of a depth coming from the beyond. It allows us to let our thoughts go, purifies and clarifies the mind, and awakens the awareness. Shiso awakens Ajna, the core of intelligence, enabling us to become aware of concepts that control us. We can say that the plant's message invites us to get rid of the aspects that create limitations for the mind, and to get rid of the residues of patterns that no longer matter in the *now*.

Properties and indications

* Depurative and detoxifying, digestive tonic, powerful anti-inflammatory: hepatic and pancreatic insufficiency and inflammation, cholesterol, diabetes, metabolic insufficiency, lithiasis, nausea, difficult digestion, lack of appetite, food intolerance, Crohn's disease, spastic colon, heavy metal intoxication, atherosclerosis, risk of heart attack, heart rhythm disorders, thrombosis, venous and lymphatic stasis

* Analgesic, powerful anti-inflammatory: chronic urogenital inflammation, inflammation of the prostate, menstrual pain and cramps, rheumatism, arthritis, muscular spasms

* Antihistaminic, anti-asthmatic, antibacterial: allergic rhinitis, asthma, chronic bronchitis, pulmonary weakness, cough

* Immune booster: immune deficiency

Suggestions

* Use this hydrosol in case of diabetes, hepatic and pancreatic insufficiency.

* Undertake a 40-day detox cure with shiso hydrosol after heavy treatments (such as chemotherapy), using 1 tbsp. in 1 litre of water (preferably hot) to be taken daily.

* The following meditation helps change bad habits:

    – Spray the shiso hydrosol in your hands and perform an auric massage.

    – Then take a sitting meditation posture.

    – Spray the hands again with the hydrosol.

    – Make 9 circles clockwise above the crown chakra.

    – 9 clockwise circles in front of the third eye.

    – 9 clockwise circles in front of the heart.

- Then place your hands on your legs, the palms touching the legs, and remain silent and observe your thoughts. Then think about the way you could step back and develop strategies to change the bad habits.

Culinary advice

❋ Spray vegetables or boiled potatoes at the end of cooking.

❋ Makes fatty sauces more digestible.

Contraindications

None.

St John's wort –*Hypericum perforatum*

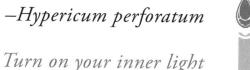

Turn on your inner light

Portrait of the plant

The French word for St John's wort is *millepertuis*, which means 'a thousand holes'. It gets this name from the small translucent glands of the common European species, *hypericum perforatum*, which has small translucent glands. When viewed through transparent sheets, these glands give the impression of a multitude of tiny perforations. St John's wort is a herbaceous plant, both annual and perennial. The flower, more or less bright yellow, has 5 petals (in rare cases 4) and many stamens.

BOTANICAL FAMILY:	Hypericaceae
PART OF THE PLANT DISTILLED:	Flowering plant
TASTE:	Bitter, soft
AROMA:	Herbaceous, earthy, warm

Principal components according to the gas chromatography of the essential oil: monoterpenes, sesquiterpenes

History and mythology

The botanical name *hypericum* in Greek means 'more than one mind'. St John's wort has traditionally been used to provide protection and chase away evil spirits. The name St John's wort (in German, *Johanniskraut*) refers to St John the Baptist who is celebrated on 24 June, the date which corresponds to the period when the plant is in blossom. St John's wort has always been celebrated as a transmitter of light. The photosensitivity of the plant confirms this quality.

Experiences with St John's wort hydrosol

Known above all for its calming and anti-inflammatory properties, the hydrosol is also a respiratory decongestant, and is often effective for respiratory allergies such as hay fever or allergy-based asthma. The Canadian author Suzanne Catty notes that a glass of water with 1 tsp. of this hydrosol, taken in winter on waking, helps fight depression associated with a lack of light.

Energy and psycho-emotional properties

It calms the nervous system, dissolving deep tensions, especially those associated with the solar plexus. It helps people ground themselves, providing a feeling of certainty and protection. It creates the link between the 1st and 3rd chakras. It purifies the aura contributing to better clarity and analysis. It balances *vata* and allows one to remain calm during turbulent periods. As a sedative, it helps in cases of sleep disorders.

Properties and indications

* Calming, purifying and anti-inflammatory at the digestive level: colic, spasms, ulcers

* Mucolytic, anti-allergic: hay fever, allergy-based asthma

* Anti-depressant, anxiolytic, sedative: depression, winter blues, emotional imbalance, lack of emotional control, troubled sleeping, state of shock, neurasthenia, susceptibility

* Healing, anti-inflammatory and cutaneous regeneration: wounds, burns, pruritus, dull complexion, sensitive skin, chapping

* Anti-inflammatory: muscular, articular and back pain, rheumatism

Suggestions

* Add St John's wort hydrosol to bath water in cases of articular and muscular pain or nervous tension.

* At night, leave a glass of water with 1 tsp. of hydrosol on the night table, drink it on waking to quickly connect the physical body and increase your morale for the day (above all in winter when it is still dark in the morning).

* For children who often have nightmares and suffer from bed-wetting, it is recommended to spray the pillow and bedroom with this hydrosol before bedtime, also adding 1 tbsp. to bath water at night.

Contraindications

According to phytotherapeutic research, St John's wort may interact with many modern-day medications. In spite of the research completed on the hydrosol, it is better to speak to your doctor if in any doubt.

Savory – *Satureja montana*

Awaken your internal power

Portrait of the plant

Savory, sometimes called *pèbre d'ase* in Provence (which literally means 'donkey's pepper'), or *poivrette* in the Swiss Valais, is a perennial and aromatic lamiaceae that we can find in the Mediterranean basin and the Balkans. It likes light, limestone soils in sunny aspects.

Botanical family:	Lamiaceae
Part of the plant distilled:	Flowering plant
Taste:	Spicy, peppery, herbaceous
Aroma:	Phenol, peppery, spicy

Principal components according to the gas chromatography of the essential oil: phenols

History and mythology

Legends say that it was one of the main plants in the magical garden of Medea. The Greeks and Romans used it as an aphrodisiac and this is why this plant was forbidden in gardens in medieval convents. This 'poison' was voluntarily used by midwives (called witches) in this period to create decoctions in order to stimulate fertility and power. For a long time savory was considered as a good luck plant in different cultures. Its name comes from the term *satyr* or the Greek *saturus*, a companion of the god Bacchus (fun-loving god in Greek mythology).

Experiences with savory hydrosol

The essential oil is renowned to be a wide spectrum antibacterial, and its hydrosol confirms this important virtue without being as aggressive and dermocaustic as the essential oil. We can observe that savory hydrosol often acts rapidly against cases of infection, and provides momentum and energy.

Energy and psycho-emotional properties

Savory increases Agni, the digestive fire, and *pitta* bioenergy. It activates the first 3 chakras, gives momentum, the ability to take the bull by the horns, the strength to act, and the ability to show courage. It is a hydrosol to use in moments of weakness, asthenic states. It helps discouraged people who feel powerless in the face of life's problems.

Properties and indications

* Antibacterial, fungicidal, virucidal: respiratory disorders, gastrointestinal infection, buccal and teeth infection, mycosis, urogenital infection, cutaneous infection

* Stimulating, hypertensive, general tonic, immuno-stimulant: hypotension, fatigue, asthenic states, nervous and physical fatigue, low libido

* Purifying at the digestive and intestinal levels: gastroenteritis, diarrhoea, intestinal candidiasis, bad breath, intestinal parasites, helicobacter pylori

Suggestions

* In cases of respiratory congestion, inhale the hydrosol.

* Spray directly in the throat or gargle for throat infections and angina/laryngitis.

* Combine savory hydrosol with rosemary verbenon hydrosol for *kapha* subjects who feel discouraged and lack motivation. Undertake a 15-day cure with 1 tsp. of each hydrosol in hot water twice a day.

* In case of intestinal candidiasis, add to colonic enemas or irrigations.

Culinary advice

* Excellent in ratatouilles, vegetable sauces and juice.

* Use as a condiment in salad dressings.

Contraindications

Pregnancy, children under 3 years old. Avoid contact with the eyes. It may burn at the mucosa level.

SPIKENARD – *Nardostachys jatamansi*

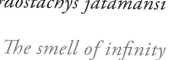

The smell of infinity

Portrait of the plant

Nardostachys jatamansi is an annual plant that grows on the slopes of the Himalayas. The large, woody and aromatic rhizomes are covered with brown-red fibres, whose thickness and number depend on the age of the plant. The rhizomes are so aromatic that their soft, captivating smell spreads in the air when they are picked. The flowers are white, pink or purple. The blossom season lasts from July to August.

BOTANICAL FAMILY:	Valerianaceae
PART OF THE PLANT DISTILLED:	Roots
TASTE:	Bitter, sweet
AROMA:	Woody, earthy, musky

Principal components according to the gas chromatography of the essential oil: sesquiterpenes, sesquiterpenols

History and mythology

Spikenard is without a doubt one of the oldest oriental perfumes and remedies. An important medicinal plant in Ayurveda, spikenard is also mentioned in ancient Egypt, in the Middle East and in ancient Rome. In the Bible, according to the Gospel of St John: 'Then Mary took about a pint of pure Spikenard, an expensive perfume; she poured it on Jesus' feet and wiped his feet with her hair. And the house was filled with the fragrance of the perfume.' Numerous ancient texts consider this plant as one of the best remedies and perfumes.

Experiences with spikenard hydrosol

It is excellent for cardiovascular problems, such as haemorrhoids and varicose veins, and also to fight stress, nervous tension, anxiety and insomnia. It facilitates awareness and reinforces confidence and clarity of mind.

Testimonial

'A 45-year-old consultant working in a financial analysis office often travelled worldwide on business. During these trips, she frequently suffered from migraine, insomnia and digestive problems and felt increasingly worn out. I suggested that she keep a small bottle of spikenard essential oil and a 30 ml hydrosol spray with her during the trips, apply several drops of the essential oil to her armpits during the trip, and spray her mouth with the hydrosol before and after meals. I also suggested that after arrival at her destination she take a shower and spray her entire body with the hydrosol, and smell the oil for 2 minutes, eyes closed, before going to bed. Since then, she feels more level-headed and serene while travelling, and the migraines have disappeared. She suffers less from jet lag and quickly re-establishes the rhythm and quality of her sleep.'

Energy and psycho-emotional properties

According to Ayurveda, spikenard is one of the most appropriate plants to balance *prana vata*, an important aspect of *vata dosha* responsible for all mental functions. It governs breathing, facilitates the circulation of *prana* (the equivalent of Qi in Chinese medicine) in the body, and sets the tone for all emotions, whether positive or negative. When *prana vata* is balanced, vital power circulates properly and we feel motivated and dynamic. If *prana vata* is dysfunctional, our immune system is weak, all cerebral functions are compromised, as such bringing on illnesses and weakened states. For these reasons, this hydrosol is effective for numerous life situations, but above all when we lack confidence and are agitated, nervous or tense.

Properties and indications

- Sedative, calming, relaxing, nervous tonic: stress, anxiety, worries, neurasthenia, nervous tension, agitation, concentration and memory problems, hyperactivity

- Hypotensor, vasodilator: haemorrhoids, varicose veins, rosacea, heavy legs, hypertension

- Diuretic, emmenagogue, antispasmodic, analgesic: menstrual pain, dysmenorrhoea, amenorrhoea, oedema

- Digestive and carminative: bloated abdomen, aerophagia, difficult digestion

Suggestions

- To reinforce *prana vata* during periods of turbulence or stress, drink a cup of hot water with 1 tsp. of hydrosol twice a day.

- To improve sleep quality, on going to bed drink a cup of hot water with 1 tsp. of spikenard hydrosol and 1 tsp. of orange blossom or Roman camomile hydrosol.

- To calm the mind before meditation or yoga, drink a cup of hot water with 1 tsp. of spikenard hydrosol. Spray the forearms with the hydrosol.

- To avoid travel problems, before your trip drink a cup of hot water with 1 tsp. of hydrosol. During long flights, bring a 30 ml bottle of hydrosol and spray the mouth and forearms from time to time.

- For haemorrhoids, varicose veins and so on: drink 1 litre of water with 2 tbsp. of spikenard hydrosol during the day (can be combined with other appropriate hydrosols). Use a compress with hydrosol on the affected zone.

- In case of menstrual pain, take 1 tsp. of hydrosol in a cup of hot water, 3 times a day.

- To treat rosacea, add spikenard hydrosol to a face mask, tone the face with this hydrosol before applying cream.

- For agitated, hyperactive, stressed children during exam periods: give 1–2 tsp. of hydrosol in water per day. Add 2–3 tbsp. of hydrosol to bath water. Spray the forearms with hydrosol.

Contraindications

None.

TEA TREE – *Melaleuca alternifolia*

Vitality and health

Portrait of the plant

A member of the myrtaceae family, *melaleuca alternifolia* is a tree that originates in Australia where it thrives in swampy areas. It can grow up to 4–6 metres in height, and its bark is papery, smooth and clear, often coming off in fine flakes. Its alternating (or supposedly alternating) leaves are needle-shaped, from 1 to 3.5 cm in length and less than 1 mm wide, persistent, hardy and bright green.

BOTANICAL FAMILY:	Myrtaceae
PART OF THE PLANT DISTILLED:	Leaves
TASTE:	Herbaceous, soft
AROMA:	Herbaceous, woody, musky

Principal components according to the gas chromatography of the essential oil: monoterpenols, monoterpenes

History and mythology

Having run out of tea during their stopovers in Australia, Captain Cook and his crew prepared an infusion with the aromatic leaves of this tree, hence its name even though it has nothing to do with traditional tea. For aboriginals, this plant has a mythical and sacred quality.

Experiences with tea tree hydrosol

As with its essential oil, the hydrosol is an important antiseptic and fungicide. The hydrosol is easier to ingest over a longer period if required to fight candidiasis and intestinal parasites. Testimonies often refer to the treatment of not only buccal but also urogenital infections.

Energy and psycho-emotional properties

The aroma of tea tree is surprising and intriguing, and it immediately connects us with our physical body and reminds us that we are embodied flesh. It re-establishes upward circulation of energy and connects the earth chakra with that of the heart. According to aboriginal legend, tea tree essential oil grew in hazardous areas to provide health care for people in the vicinity. This reminds us of the strength of Mother Earth and that this general antiseptic provides protection. It dissolves away bitterness, unhealthy fears fed by those around us, and guilt.

Properties and indications

* Antibacterial, virucidal, fungicidal: mycosis, acne, dermatosis, wounds, buccal infections, gingivitis, mouth sores, periodontitis, conjunctivitis, urogenital infections, respiratory disorders

* Metabolic stimulant: hypothyroidism, heavy digestion

* Lymphatic and blood stimulant: venous and lymphatic stasis, haemorrhoids, cellulite, thrombosis, varicose veins

* Nervous tonic and immune system stimulant: fragile nerves, fatigue, immune system weakness

Suggestions

* Rinsing teeth with 1 tsp. of tea tree hydrosol in a glass of water prevents tooth decay, and inflamed and bleeding gums. Spray the mouth regularly when installing a dental apparatus.

* To disinfect a child's injury, simply spray the wound with the hydrosol.

* Use as a tonic or in a mask for acne.

* In cases of vaginal mycosis, use it for vaginal douches (including during pregnancy): 1 tsp. of hydrosol in 100 ml of water and apply a compress to the genital area.

* As protection against mycosis, spray the feet before and after going to the gym or pool changing room.

* Gargle with tea tree, savory or thyme thymol hydrosol in cases of laryngitis.

* A 7-day cure with tea tree hydrosol taken internally, also using the essential oil on the soles of the feet, can help people who feel overwhelmed by work. It helps cultivate the conviction of having the vital strength to fulfil their mission.

Contraindications

None.

THYME LINALOOL – *Thymus vulgaris linaloliferum*

Sweetly heal

Portrait of the plant

Thymus vulgaris is a small perennial subshrub, bushy and very aromatic, 7–30 cm in height, which grows throughout the Mediterranean basin and also in the Americas. It likes dry limestone soil and direct sun.

BOTANICAL FAMILY:	Lamiaceae
PART OF THE PLANT DISTILLED:	Whole plant
TASTE:	Herbaceous, soft
AROMA:	Soft, herbaceous

Principal components according to the gas chromatography of the essential oil: monoterpenols

History and mythology

In Greek, the word *thymus* (or *thumo*) means courage or transformation by fire. In ancient Greece, when leaving for battle the heads of warriors would be decorated with a crown of thyme to help them confront their enemy with courage. To this day in certain regions of Greece, they say that someone 'smells like thyme' to designate them as someone special, extraordinary and fearless. Greek doctors, including Hippocrates, considered thyme as one of the main medicinal plants for treating various pathologies (gynaecological, urinary, pulmonary problems) and during childbirth.

Experiences with thyme linalool hydrosol

Thyme quietly activates the immune system. It is a sweet hydrosol but a very efficient disinfectant and is particularly recommended for children and babies. It is also often used for skin infections.

Energy and psycho-emotional properties

It is particularly recommended for people who absorb 'collective viruses', i.e. those who easily become sick during epidemics, and also those who easily adopt collective ideas and attitudes without questioning them. Thyme linalool hydrosol can be used as a purifying aura spray.

Properties and indications

* Neurotonic and nervous system balancer: asthenic states, nervous fatigue, stress

* Immune booster: immune deficiency, convalescence

* Antibacterial, virucidal, fungicidal: buccal infections, mouth sores, gingivitis, respiratory infections, intestinal infections, urogenital infections, colitis, enterocolitis, mycosis

* Important cutaneous disinfectant: impetigo, wounds, mycosis, boils, acne

Suggestions

* In cases of immune deficiency, add 1 tbsp. to 1 litre of water to drink during the day as a 40-day cure.

* In cases of impetigo or other cutaneous infections, spray the affected zone several times a day in combination with geranium hydrosol.

* Add 1 tsp. to a baby's bath water as protection during the cold and flu season.

* Spray a baby's bottom to help with nappy rash.

Culinary advice

❁ Gives a soft and herbaceous note to soups, vegetables and sauces.

❁ Sophisticated for ice cream, sherbets and other desserts.

Contraindications

None.

Thyme thymol – *Thymus vulgaris thymoliferum*

A booster

Portrait of the plant

Same profile as thyme linalool with the following differences:

TASTE:	Characteristic of thyme, herbaceous, spicy
AROMA:	Hot, spicy, herbaceous

Principal components according to the gas chromatography of the essential oil: phenols

Experiences with thyme thymol hydrosol

This is one of the best antibacterial hydrosols, and is particularly recommended for respiratory and urogenital infections. It boosts and transmits power and strength. During convalescence, it helps build strength, and supports a fragile immune system.

Testimonial

'I suggest it in cases of acute cystitis, combining it with equal parts of savory and cinnamon hydrosols and adding 2 tbsp. to 1 litre of hot water to drink during the day. The following essential oils can also be applied to the lower part of the stomach at the same time: ginger, sandalwood and tea tree. With this regime, the symptoms quickly disappear and recuperation is rapid. In most cases these steps avoid the need for antibiotics.'

Energy and psycho-emotional properties

This energy booster helps during periods of weakness when overcome by fear. It helps 'take the bull by the horns' when one feels like fleeing a conflict. It dilates the 1st chakra and transmits the necessary force to fight against an inferiority complex and feelings of frustration.

Properties and indications

<ul>
<li>Antibacterial, virucidal, fungicidal: wounds, dermatosis, buccal infection, mycosis, acne, colds, intestinal and respiratory infection, urogenital infection</li>
<li>Immune booster: immune deficiency, convalescence</li>
</ul>

Suggestions

<ul>
<li>For colds, sinus infections and bronchitis, add 2 tbsp. of thyme thymol hydrosol to 1 litre of boiling water and inhale.</li>
<li>In cases of urinary infection, drink a cup of hot water with 1 tsp. of thyme thymol hydrosol every hour.</li>
<li>Gargle or spray the throat to help with a sore throat.</li>
</ul>

Culinary advice

<ul>
<li>Gives a Mediterranean taste to ratatouille and tomato sauces.</li>
</ul>

Contraindications

Pregnancy, children.

LEMON VERBENA – *Lippia citriodora*

Change for the better

Portrait of the plant

Lemon verbena is a small aromatic shrub that can reach 2 metres in height and grows wild in South America. *Lippia* (or also *Aloysia*) *citriodora* is a shrub cultivated for its very aromatic leaves, to add aroma to some dishes and to prepare infusions and liqueurs. It is a plant originally from the Andes region in South America (Peru, Bolivia, Chile and Argentina) where it grows at 2000–3000 metres.

BOTANICAL FAMILY:	Verbenaceae
PART OF THE PLANT DISTILLED:	Leaves
TASTE:	Soft, slightly lemony
AROMA:	Lemony, flowery, fruity

Principal components according to the gas chromatography of the essential oil: aldehydes

History and mythology

Verbena was associated with the goddess Isis and the planet Sirius. The Romans referred to this plant as 'Isis Plant', 'Sacred Plant', 'Juno's Tear', 'Hercules' Plant' and also 'Mercury's Blood'. The stems and branches of this delicate shrub were used for making ceremonial crowns. The Latin word *verbenaca* means 'sacred branch' or 'magical wand'. Venus was always decorated with myrtle and verbena. The Greeks gave it many names, and used it for their ceremonies as well as in medicine. The Gallic druids used it for making prophecies and to show clairvoyance.

Experiences with lemon verbena hydrosol

The essential oil is considered to be a major anti-inflammatory and its hydrosol confirms this property. It is very effective at the psycho-emotional level, dissolving fear, and being invigorating and deeply relaxing at the same time, while helping one to balance extreme emotions.

Energy and psycho-emotional properties

Verbena acts like morning dew. The new day starts: 'We are relaxed, we don't know what the day holds for us, everything is new and unknown, but we're not worried.' Verbena is fresh but never cold, calm without tiring. Verbena is probably one of the most powerful remedies for fighting depression. It opens us to new things, dilates the heart chakra and brings joy and optimism.

Properties and indications

- Major anti-inflammatory and spasmolytic: skin and mucus inflammation, buccal inflammation, intestinal inflammation, menstrual spasm, colic

- Stimulates liver, pancreatic, intestinal and thyroid functions: hypothyroidism, hepatic and pancreatic insufficiency, difficult digestion, premenstrual syndrome

- Neurotonic, sedative and anti-depressant: gloom, nervous fatigue, depression, fear, lack of motivation, insomnia, lethargy, worry, lack of confidence

- Eases childbirth, according to Latin American shamans

- Slightly diuretic effect: during weight gain, above all before periods

Suggestions

- In cases of bad mood, gloom, grief or depression linked to seasonal change, use the hydrosol as an auric and air spray; drink 1 litre of water with 1 tbsp. of hydrosol daily; add 2 tbsp. of hydrosol to bath water.

- Combine with rosemary verbenon, shiso or ledum hydrosol for purification cures.

- Three times a day drink a glass of hot water with 1 tsp. to ease childbirth and dissolve fears. Start 2 weeks before due date.

- Take a cup of hot water with 1 tsp. of hydrosol after a heavy meal.

- For skin infections or inflammation due to psycho-emotional causes, spray the skin and drink 1 tbsp. in 1 litre of water a day.

- Use in combination with peppermint hydrosol for fresh breath.

- Use as an excellent ambiance spray when the atmosphere is 'electric'.

Culinary advice

- Gives a divine lemony taste to risotto and mushroom recipes.

- Spray fruit salads and sherbets.

- Add to relaxing teas.

- Delicious in fruit juices and smoothies – refreshing and exhilarating.

- Spray green vegetables.

Contraindications

Pregnancy.

VETIVER – *Vetiveria zizanoides*

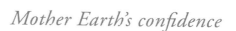

Mother Earth's confidence

Portrait of the plant

Vetiver is a perennial bunchgrass of the poaceae family. It shares many morpho-logical characteristics with other fragrant grasses, such as lemongrass or palmarosa. Vetiver grows to 150 cm high and forms clumps as wide. Under favourable conditions, the erect culms can reach 3 metres in height. The stems are tall, and the leaves are long, thin and rather rigid. The flowers are brownish-purple. Unlike most grasses, which form horizontally spreading, mat-like root systems, vetiver's roots grow downward, 2–4 metres in depth. Vetiver originates in India and is today widely cultivated in tropical regions of the world as Haiti, Indonesia and Reunion.

BOTANICAL FAMILY:	Grasses (poaceae)
PART OF THE PLANT DISTILLED:	Roots
TASTE:	Soft, slightly bitter, fresh
AROMA:	Woody, earthy

Principal components according to the gas chromatography of the essential oil: sesquiterpenes, sesquiterpernols

History and mythology

Vetiver's earthy aroma has been much appreciated since time immemorial, not only in India but also in Java where it is known as *Akar wangi*, which means 'aromatic roots'. Ayurveda proclaims its medicinal virtues for treating circulatory problems. In India, newlyweds receive a balm containing vetiver to cement their relationship, make them fertile, and as a benediction for the couple's prosperity.

Experiences with vetiver hydrosol

The hydrosol works as a circulatory tonic and its grounding properties provide reassurance. *Vata* and *pitta* types can act and think in a calmer fashion.

Energy and psycho-emotional properties

Vetiver, as an essential oil or hydrosol, brings the certainty that abundance is a natural state that each person deserves. It roots us, and helps us develop trust in Mother Earth. This trust brings on the ability to develop concrete long-term projects and strong relationships. It is particularly useful for people who are obsessed about security, and suffer because they are overwhelmed by fear.

Properties and indications

* Circulatory and lymphatic tonic, firming, hydrating: asphyxiated skin, rosacea, dry skin, cellulite, thrombosis, hives, varicose veins, haemorrhoids, coronary arteritis, vascularity

* Emmenagogue, endocrinal stimulant: amenorrhoea, dysmenorrhoea, premenopausal syndrome

* Digestive, pancreatic and hepatic stimulant: hepatic and pancreatic congestion, difficult digestion, aerophagia

* Calming and sedative: mental agitation, fear of loss, worries, mental dispersion, anger, excess *vata*, instability, excessive need for security, difficulty in delegating, anxiety in the face of the unknown

* Immune booster and nervous tonic: asthenic states, immune deficiency, digestive weakness

Suggestions

- Use as a tonic or cutaneous spray in cases of rosacea, flabby, wrinkled and asphyxiated skin. Combined with frankincense hydrosol, it intensifies the anti-wrinkle effect.

- Sitz baths and compresses create a soothing effect for varicose veins or haemorrhoids. Also drink 1 litre of water with 2 tbsp. of hydrosol a day in combination with other suitable hydrosols.

- To improve sleep, before bed drink a cup of hot water with 1 tsp. of vetiver hydrosol and 1 tsp. of orange blossom or Roman camomile hydrosol.

- In cases of worry and mental agitation, drink a cup of hot water with 1 tsp. of hydrosol. Spray the forearms with the hydrosol.

- Bloating and difficult digestion linked to nervousness and mental agitation can be soothed by drinking a cup of hot water with 1 tsp. of hydrosol before meals. A hot compress on the belly with hydrosol also soothes a sensitive stomach.

- Spray reactive skin before applying natural creams.

- Spray wounds that are slow to heal, and varicose ulcers.

Culinary advice

- Gives a woody taste to desserts and makes them easier to digest.

- Increases the anti-*pitta* aspect in lhassi and milkshakes.

- Gives a sophisticated and woody note to vanilla or hazelnut ice cream.

Contraindications

Pregnancy.

Vitex – *Agnus castus*

Accept and act

Portrait of the plant

Originally from the Mediterranean basin, vitex, also known as chasteberry or chaste tree, is a perennial bush with palm-like leaves. In the summer, it is full of small violet flowers that transform into seeds used for distillation. The whole plant is very aromatic.

Botanical family:	Valerianaceae
Part of the plant distilled:	Berries
Taste:	Bitter
Aroma:	Woody, earthy

Principal components according to the gas chromatography of the essential oil: oxides, monoterpenes, sesquiterpenes

History and mythology

Vitex (in German, *mönchspfeffer* meaning 'monk's pepper') is renowned for reducing male sexual drive, which is why, during the Middle Ages, monasteries cultivated this wild pepper and mixed it with food. Just like the monks who used it to control their carnal desires, Greek women gave it to their husbands when they didn't want the family to grow. Even today, some Italian monasteries cover the ground with vitex branches when novices first arrive.

Experiences with vitex hydrosol

Vitex is known for its progesterone-like effects and has shown itself to be useful in premenstrual syndrome, premenopausal stages, or with overly abundant periods.

Energy and psycho-emotional properties

Vitex calms irritability and helps overcome problems linked to change. It lightens the change process necessary for personal evolution and helps us to work through these periods more effectively. It calms and harmonises emotions, drains excess heat accumulated in the liver, kidneys and the urogenital tract. In this way, it brings on a feeling of lightness. It drives energy from the 1st to the 6th chakra.

Properties and indications

- Progesterone-like, important hormonal balancer, uterine and ovarian regenerator: menopause problems, premenstrual syndrome, hormone-based migraines, dysmenorrhoea, amenorrhoea, weight gain (linked to menopausal disorders), haemorrhagic periods

- Nervous and emotional balancer especially linked to hormonal fluctuations: neurasthenia, irritability, susceptibility

- Appetite regulator: digestive troubles and excess appetite linked to menstrual problems

- Skin purifier: acne outbreak before periods

- Uterine and ovarian regenerator: ovarian cysts, fibroids

Suggestions

- Drink 1 litre of water with 1 tbsp. of hydrosol a week before and during periods to prevent premenstrual syndrome and acne outbreaks.

* For menopausal problems, drink 1 litre of water with 1 tbsp. of hydrosol and add 1–2 tbsp. to bath water. It can be combined with other suitable hydrosols.

Contraindications

Hormone-dependent cancers, children.

Yarrow – *Achillea millefolium*
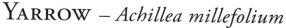

Creating balance between opposition

Portrait of the plant

Yarrow is a herbaceous plant 60–90 cm high, perennial and very widespread. The whole plant looks like an umbelliferous. The cut leaves probably influenced the Latin name, as *millefolium* means 1000 leaves.

BOTANICAL FAMILY:	Asteraceae
PART OF THE PLANT DISTILLED:	Flowers and whole plant
TASTE:	Soft, earthy, a bit acidic
AROMA:	Woody, soft, slightly reminiscent of hay

Principal components according to the gas chromatography of the essential oil: oxides, monoterpenes

History and mythology

Achilles, the warrior from the Greek tragedy *The Iliad*, supposedly used it to heal the wounds of his comrade Telephos during the Battle of Troy. Hippocrates proclaimed the merits of yarrow, notably for cardiovascular problems and in particular for haemorrhoids and varicose veins. In the Mediterranean basin, it is still known today under many names such as 'cut grass', 'nosebleed' or 'carpenter weed'. In ancient China, it was venerated for its yin and yang qualities, which were supposed to be brought together in perfect harmony – firmness and hardness for the outside of the stem, the suppleness and emptiness for the interior.

Experiences with yarrow hydrosol

Yarrow hydrosol has often worked well for gynaecological disorders including hormonal imbalances, fibroids, menopausal problems, premenstrual syndrome and painful menstruation. It should be used when a woman is in a situation of change or crisis (particularly effective after childbirth, in cases of separation, professional change, or when the children leave home). Yarrow, whether essential oil or hydrosol, is also one of the most recommended plants for neuralgia. It soothes pain and balances the nervous system by transmitting a feeling of certainty.

Testimonial

'A midwife's testimonial: 'Just after the birth I spray the perineum of women (particularly in cases of episiotomies and tearing) with a blend of equal parts of yarrow, cistus and everlasting hydrosols. Then the wound heals well and quickly. I spray 2–3 times a day and I then dry it with a hair dryer.'

Energy and psycho-emotional properties

Yarrow helps us better to understand our surroundings, opposing polarities, and people with whom communication is difficult. It supports adaptation to new situations, and changes during periods of transition. It also enhances understanding between men and women. It is also a good stabilising influence during times of change such as mid-life crisis, menopause and challenges at work. Sometimes the hydrosol acts as a sedative, especially when insomnia occurs as a result of conflict or stress.

Properties and indications

- Hormonal balancing for women: menopausal problems, premenstrual syndrome, abundant menstruation, fibroids, myomas, painful periods

- Digestive, spasmolytic: difficult digestion, colic, constipation

- Anti-haemorrhagic: abundant menstruation, varicose ulcers, cuts (as a compress), bleeding haemorrhoids (sitz bath), endometriosis (ingestion and sitz bath)

- Expectorant: bronchitis, cough

- Analgesic: headaches, rheumatism

- Circulatory and lymphatic stimulant: cellulite, heavy legs, varicose veins

- Healing agent: varicose ulcers, wounds

Suggestions

- For repeated headaches, crisis or coping with change, take a 40-day cure with yarrow hydrosol (twice a day, 1 tsp. in a glass of warm water after meals).

- A sitz bath enriched with 1 tbsp. of yarrow hydrosol soothes haemorrhoids, pelvic pain and genital itching.

- A vaginal douche – 200 ml of water with 1 tbsp. of Yarrow hydrosol – helps with fibroids and haemorrhagic periods.

- Compresses with yarrow hydrosol soothe irritated skin, rosacea, varicose veins and heavy legs, but also painful zones caused by rheumatism.

- For wounds, it is ideal for cleaning and to stop bleeding.

- For eczema, hives and itching, spraying the zone calms and refreshes.

- For feet with pressure ulcers or calluses, foot baths are calming and soothing.

- In cases of bronchitis and a cough, drink a glass of warm water with 1–2 tsp.; gargle several times a day.

- To support renal function, use as a mild diuretic: 1 glass of warm water with 1 tsp. of yarrow hydrosol 3 times a day.

Contraindications

Pregnancy.

YLANG YLANG – *Cananga odorata*

Let it go, let it come

Portrait of the plant

Ylang ylang is a tree with persistent foliage which when farmed is generally trimmed to a height of 2–3 metres, but can attain 25–30 metres in the wild, with a generously spread crown. The petals give off a penetrating, spicy smell reminiscent of carnation, narcissus and jasmine. The petals, which start white, become greenish before turning yellow with a red base. Flowering takes place throughout the year but is more abundant during hot and humid periods.

BOTANICAL FAMILY:	Anonaceae
PART OF THE PLANT DISTILLED:	Flowers
TASTE:	Soft, slightly acidic
AROMA:	Flowery, suave, reminiscent of jasmine

Principal components according to the gas chromatography of the essential oil: oxides, monoterpenes, sesquiterpenes

History and mythology

The term *ylang ylang* comes from the Philippines where it is called *alang-ilang* in reference to the flowers that dance in the wind. Filipinos traditionally macerated ylang ylang flowers in coconut oil to produce *boori-boori*, a universal ointment that reduced fevers and infections, nourished skin and hair, and provided protection from the sun and sea salt. In Indonesia *ylang ylang* means 'the flower of flowers' and in fact there is no softer fragrance. To this day, they cover newlyweds' beds with ylang ylang petals.

Experiences with ylang ylang hydrosol

The sensual and exhilarating aroma enhances creativity. The hydrosol promotes relaxation, calms the turbulent mind and dissolves resistance and rigidity. It invites the mind to let go of worries, dare to dream, and live life to the full.

Energy and psycho-emotional properties

Ylang ylang awakens passion and the desire to take full advantage of all aspects of life. Like its essential oil, the hydrosol increases intuition, creativity and the ability to communicate. It dilates Svadhistana, the 2nd chakra, and in so doing helps introverted people open up. It awakens sensuality and helps one feel more passion, joy and love without fear or guilt. It lightens and changes one's viewpoint when the mind has become rigid and resistant.

Properties and indications

* Hydrating, soothing and antiseptic tonic for the skin: mature and asphyxiated skin, psoriasis, eczema, hives, dandruff, wrinkles, dermatosis, mycosis

* Anti-depressant, sedative, anxiolytic: depression, stress, anxiety, mental rigidity, dark ideas, shock, sorrow, inability to forget about worries, doubts, difficulty communicating

* Hypotensor and vasodilator: hypertension, thrombosis, varicose veins, rosacea, palpitations, arrhythmia, tachycardia

* Aphrodisiac: impotence, frigidity, lack of joy and lightness, inability to feel pleasure, lack of passion

Suggestions

* Spray in the bedroom and on the body before making love.

* Spray the face, wrists and add to bath water after a busy and stressful day.

- Drink 1 litre of water with 1 tbsp. of hydrosol a day in cases of hypertension (can be combined with other suitable hydrosols).

- If communication is difficult as a result of introversion and shyness, and when the feeling of joy and pleasure is absent, undertake a 40-day cure drinking 1 litre of water with 1 tbsp. of hydrosol daily while spraying the face and wrists with the hydrosol. At the same time, smell the essential oil.

Culinary advice

- Gives an exotic note to salads and fruit juices.

Contraindications

None.

TREATMENT SUGGESTIONS

The proposed treatment suggestions are aimed at both the preventive and curative aspects of diseases. The hydrosols can be used alone or combined with other therapeutic approaches, and can be used safely in conjunction with other treatment regimes in aromatherapy and phytotherapy.

It goes without saying that close reading of this book will enable you to modify any one of the formulas and create your own concoctions. Follow your intuition while respecting the necessary safety guidelines. Also remember that no book can replace the advice of an experienced professional.

The therapeutic advice given in this section is based on reports from therapists in many different fields, and also people who simply love hydrosols (many of their testimonies are found in the descriptions). However, please bear in mind that every individual is unique and requires an original and personalised approach.

Furthermore, it is a good idea to consult the individual plant descriptions before creating a preparation in order to confirm the properties of each plant and consider any possible contraindications.

Of course, the advice of a doctor or an experienced therapist is important if symptoms persist.

Experience also shows that we are more likely to continue with a treatment if the blend tastes good and is enjoyable to take. Take this into account. When you create a blend, start with a small quantity so you can modify it if necessary.

Abbreviations

Tsp. = teaspoon
Tbsp. = tablespoon
ml = millilitre
QS = quantum satis (amount which is needed)

EO = essential oil
HS = hydrosol
CO = carrier oil

It may be that the reader will be surprised by certain formulas of pure essential oils. The suggestions come mostly from the experiences of Swiss practitioners and therapists. Aromatherapy and hydrosol therapy in our country are influenced by the French school of aromatherapy but with a holistic and often a spiritual vision. If you are not comfortable with the use of pure essential oils blends, you can, of course, dilute them with a carrier oil. However, we have also observed that the use of pure essential oils (for example under the soles of the feet where the skin is less sensitive) can accelerate the healing process especially in case of infection when the bacteria or virus multiply in large speed.

Approximate measurements of essential oils
0.25 ml EO = 5 drops
0.5 ml EO = 10 drops
1 ml EO = 20 drops
2 ml EO = 40 drops
3 ml EO = 60 drops
4 ml EO = 80 drops
5 ml EO = 100 drops
6 ml EO = 120 drops

1. Hydrosol therapy for the respiratory system

Angina (see throat infection)

Aphonia
Spray the throat or gargle several times a day with the following mix:

HS Winter savory/*Satureja montana*	30 ml
HS Cinnamon bark/*Cinnamomum verum*	30 ml
HS Bergamot/*Citrus bergamia*	40 ml

Allergy-based asthma

The following blend can also be used for prevention. It is important that a medical doctor follows up on the treatment.

HS Kewra/*Pandanus odoratum*	25 ml
HS Blue camomile/*Camomilla matricaria*	50 ml
HS Shiso/*Perilla frutescens*	25 ml

Spray in the mouth several times in a row in case of attack.

Drink a cup of hot water with 1 tsp. of the mix 2–3 times a day.

Bronchitis and cough

HS Myrtle/*Myrtus communis*	50 ml
HS Eucalyptus/*Eucalyptus globulus*	25 ml
HS Ravintsara/*Cinnamomum camphora*	50 ml
HS Cypress/*Cupressus sempervirens*	50 ml
HS Scots pine/*Pinus sylvestris*	75 ml
HS Thyme thymol/*Thymus vulgaris thymoliferum*	50 ml

Drink 1 tsp. in a cup of hot water before meals, depending on the situation. Continue treatment 3–4 days after symptoms disappear.

Take a hot bath with 3 tbsp. of the mix.

Externally:

EO Myrtle/*Myrtus communis*	1 ml
EO Cypress/*Cupressus sempervirens*	2 ml
EO Brazilian pepper/*Schinus terebentifolius*	1 ml
EO Sweet fennel/*Foeniculum vulgaris dulce*	1 ml
EO Saro/*Cinnamosma fragrans*	2 ml
EO Rosalina/*Melaleuca ericifolia*	1 ml

Massage the thorax, the upper back and soles of the feet 4 times a day depending on the situation. Continue 3–4 days after symptoms disappear.

Cold and flu-like states

HS Scots pine/*Pinus sylvestris*	50 ml
HS Rosemary verbenon/*Rosmarinus verbenoniferum*	50 ml
HS Thyme linalool/*Thymus vulg. Linaloliferum*	50 ml
HS Myrtle/*Myrtus communis*	50 ml

Add 1 tsp. to a cup of hot water and drink 3–5 times a day, based on the situation.

HS Scots pine/*Pinus sylvestris*	25 ml
HS Myrtle/*Myrtus communis*	25 ml
HS Thyme linalool/*Thymus vulg. linaloliferum*	50 ml
HS Tea tree/*Melaleuca alternifolia*	25 ml

Use as a nasal spray several times a day based on the situation.

For inhaling:
Place a few drops of Scots pine, *eucalyptus radiata*, peppermint, cajuput, niaouli or black spruce essential oils on a tissue (choose 2–3 from the list) and inhale.

Externally:
Massage the thorax, forehead and sinuses with a couple of drops of the essential oils mentioned above.

Other recommended hydrosols for cold and flu-like states: rosemary verbenon, ravintsara, bay laurel, savory, cinnamon, thyme thymol, juniper, cypress, eucalyptus globulus.

Hay fever

HS St John's wort/*Hypericum perforatum*	100 ml
HS Blue camomile/*Chamomilla matricaria*	100 ml

Add 1 tbsp. to 1.5 litres of water and drink during the day. Begin 2–3 weeks before the appearance of first symptoms and during the season.

Myrtle, Scots pine and basil hydrosols can also be used to soothe symptoms.

Spray itchy eyes with myrtle hydrosol.

Prana/Chi

The following blend improves the circulation of prana/chi (vital power, breath). It can be used as an auric spray, as a drink (1 tsp. in a cup of hot water), in bath water (3–4 tbsp.) or as a compress on the chest in case of respiratory difficulty or congestion.

HS Shiso/*Perilla frutescens*	20 ml
HS Angelica/*Angelica archangelica*	20 ml
HS Blue camomile/*Chamomilla matricaria*	50 ml
HS Eucalyptus/*Eucalyptus globulus*	30 ml
HS Everlasting/*Helichrysum italicum*	20 ml
HS Kewra/*Pandanus odoratissimus*	50 ml
HS St John's wort/*Hypericum perforatum*	50 ml
HS Thyme linalool/*Thymus vulgaris linalool*	50 ml
HS Bergamot/*Citrus aurantium bergamia*	110 ml

Sinus infections

HS Myrtle/*Myrtus communis*	25 ml
HS Rosemary verbenon/*Rosmarinus verbenoniferum*	25 ml
HS Ravintsara/*Cinnamomum camphora*	50 ml
HS Scots pine/*Pinus sylvestris*	50 ml
HS Helichrysum/*Helichrysum italicum*	25 ml

Use as a nasal spray several times a day.

Add 1 tsp. of the mix to a cup of hot water and drink 3–4 times a day. Continue 1 week after symptoms disappear (for a more antibacterial and warming effect, 1 tsp. of savory, cinnamon or thyme thymol can be added to the hot water).

Inhale with 1 litre of water, 1 tbsp. of the hydrosol blend and 3 drops of eucalyptus globulus or radiata essential oil.

Externally:
Apply rosemary verbenon, Roman camomile or helichrysum essential oil on the sinuses towards the nose; continue treatment based on situation.

Throat infection, Angina, Laryngitis

Spray the throat with savory hydrosol and/or thyme thymol hydrosol.

Externally:

EO Tea tree/*Melaleuca alternifolia*	1.0 ml
EO Saro/*Cinnamosma fragrans*	1.0 ml
EO Scots pine/*Pinus sylvestris*	2.0 ml
EO Sandalwood/*Santalum album*	0.5 ml

Rub soles of the feet, the neck and chest twice a day.

To protect the immune system during cold season

Undertake a cure with ravintsara, Scots pine, thyme linalool, geranium and frankincense hydrosols. Or regularly drink these hydrosols as a tea, adding 1 tsp. to a cup of hot water.

2. Hydrosol therapy for the digestive and metabolic system

Aerophagia

Antispasmodic and digestive:
HS Basil/*Ocimum basilicum*
HS Cinnamon bark/*Cinnamomum verum*

Add 1 tsp. of each to a cup of hot water and drink before meals or as needed. For other recommended hydrosols see 'Digestive' in the therapeutic index.

Appetite (lack of)

According to Ayurveda and Chinese medicine, it is toxic to eat if you are not really hungry. This is symptomatic of a weak digestive fire. The following treatment can also be effective in case of loss of appetite during chemotherapy.

HS Bergamot/*Citrus bergamia*	50 ml
HS Cinnamon bark/*Cinnamomum verum*	50 ml

Add 1 tsp. of the blend to 1.5 litres of water and drink during the day, or drink a cup of hot water with 1 tsp. of the blend before meals.

Appetite (excessive)

HS Champak/*Michelia alba*	50 ml
HS Sandalwood/*Santalum album*	50 ml
HS Rose/*Rosa damascene*	50 ml
HS Coriander/*Coriandrum sativum*	50 ml

Add 1 tbsp. of the mix to 1.5 litres of water and drink during the day for 21 days. Stop for 9 days and then restart if necessary.

If the excessive appetite is due to hormonal imbalance:

HS Sage/*Salvia officinalis*	50 ml
HS Clary sage/*Salvia sclarea*	50 ml
HS Geranium/*Pelargonium asperum*	50 ml
HS Lemon verbena/*Lippia citriodora*	50 ml

Add 1 tbsp. of the mix to 1.5 litres of water and drink during the day for 21 days. Stop for 9 days, then restart if necessary.

Biliary and pancreatic insufficiency

Internally:

HS Angelica/*Angelica archangelica*	20 ml
HS Sweet linalool basil/*Ocimum basilicum*	60 ml
HS Cinnamon bark/*Cinnamomum verum*	40 ml
HS Geranium/*Pelargonium asperum*	60 ml
HS Kewra/*Pandanus odoratus*	20 ml
HS Ledum/*Rhododendron groenlandicum*	20 ml
HS Clary sage/*Salvia sclarea*	60 ml
HS Lemon verbena/*Lippia citriodora*	120 ml

Add 1 tbsp. to 1.5 litres of water and drink during the day for 40 days. Stop for 10 days and restart if necessary.

Cholesterol

Very effective with quick results:

HS Carrot/*Daucus carota*	100 ml
HS Geranium/*Pelargonium asperum*	200 ml
HS Everlasting/*Helichrysum italicum*	100 ml
HS Shiso/*Perilla frutescens*	100 ml
HS Ledum/*Rhododendron groenlandicum*	100 ml
HS Bergamot/*Citrus bergamia*	200 ml

Add 2 tbsp. to 1 litre of water and drink during the day. Undertake a 40-day cure and repeat if necessary.

Cirrhosis (adjuvant)

Hepatic regeneration:

HS Ledum/*Rhododendron groenlandicum*	50 ml
HS Shiso/*Perilla frutescens*	50 ml
HS Carrot/*Daucus carota*	25 ml
HS Everlasting/*Helichrysum italicum*	25 ml
HS Peppermint/*Mentha piperita*	100 ml
HS Rose/*Rosa damascena*	100 ml

Add 1 tbsp. of the blend to 1.5 litres of water and drink during the day for several months, depending on the situation.

Colitis

HS Yarrow/*Achillea millefolium*
HS Basil/*Ocimum basilicum*
HS Roman camomile/*Chamaemelum nobile*
HS Cinnamon/*Cinnamomum verum*
HS Shiso/*Perilla frutescens*

HS Bergamot/*Citrus bergamia*

HS Marjoram/*Origanum majorana*

HS Rosemary verbenon/*Rosmarinus verbenoniferum*

HS Sandalwood/*Santalum album*

Choose 1–3 of these hydrosols and add 1 tsp. of each to a cup of hot water, and drink every 30 minutes based on the situation.

Use hot compresses on the painful zone with the same hydrosols.

Apply locally on the painful zone essential oils such as marjoram, sandalwood, lavender or sweet fennel, every 30 minutes based on the situation.

Constipation

HS Bergamot/*Citrus bergamia*	50 ml
HS Yarrow/*Achillea millefolium*	25 ml
HS Basil/*Ocimum basilicum*	25 ml

Mix 1 tsp. of the blend with a cup of hot water, 3 tbsp. of apple juice, a bit of honey and a drop of mandarin EO. Drink before meals for 21 days or as needed.

Use a hot compress with 2–3 tbsp. of the blend on the stomach.

Externally (in addition):

EO Ginger/*Zingiber officinalis*	0.25 ml
EO Sandalwood/*Santalum album*	0.25 ml

Massage the stomach.

Crohn's disease

HS Lemon verbena/*Lippia citriodora*	100 ml
HS Cistus/*Cistus ladaniferus*	50 ml
HS Shiso/*Perilla frutescens*	50 ml
HS Roman camomile/*Chamaemelum nobile*	100 ml
HS Frankincense/*Boswellia carterii*	50 ml
HS Orange blossom/*Citrus aurantium (blossoms)*	50 ml

Add 1 tsp. to a cup of hot water and drink before meals.

EO Lemon verbena/*Lippia citriodora*	0.5 ml
EO Neroli/*Citrus aurantium (blossoms)*	0.5 ml
EO Cistus/*Cistus ladaniferus*	3.0 ml
EO Roman camomile/*Chamaemelum nobile*	1.0 ml
CO *Calophyllum inophyllum* QS	20.0 ml

Apply to the lower stomach and back, twice a day based on the situation.

Diabetes (adjuvant)

HS Angelica/*Angelica archangelica*	50 ml
HS Shiso/*Perilla frutescens*	50 ml
HS Geranium/*Pelargonium asperum*	100 ml
HS Verbena/*Lippia citriodora*	100 ml
HS Helichrysum/*Helichrysum italicum*	25 ml
HS Scots pine/*Pinus sylvestris*	25 ml

Add 1 tsp. of the blend to a cup of hot water morning, noon and night, to take before meals for 2–3 months. Stop for 1 month, then restart.

Digestive spasms

HS Marjoram/*Origanum majorana*
HS Basil/*Ocimum basilicum*
HS Roman camomile/*Chamaemelum nobile*

Add 1 tsp. of each to a cup of hot water; repeat if necessary.

Hot compress on the stomach (soak a towel in hot water and add 1–4 tbsp. of each).

Take a hot bath with 1 tbsp. of each.

Excessive need for sugar

Hydrosols such as champaca, coriander, kewra, geranium, palmarosa or rose soothe the *pitta* bioenergy and can diminish the need for sugar. Add 1 tbsp. of

1 or 2 of the above hydrosols to 1 litre of water and drink during the day. You can also drink it as a tea in a cup of hot water with 1 tsp.

Gastric acidity

HS Coriander/*Coriandrum sativum*	50 ml
HS Roman camomile/*Chamaemelum nobile*	25 ml
HS Peppermint/*Mentha piperita*	50 ml
HS Basil/*Ocimum basilicum*	25 ml
HS Angelica/*Angelica archangelica*	25 ml

Add 1 tsp. of the blend to a cup of hot water and drink 2–5 times a day, based on the situation. At the same time, diminish acidic foods, such as sugar, alcohol and coffee.

If the gastric acidity continues, a liver and pancreas detox can also be effective. (See the relevant hydrosols in the therapeutic index.) In case of isolated or rare symptoms, a hot compress on the stomach and a cup of hot water with 1 tsp. of the first 3 hydrosols mentioned above can be sufficient.

Hepatic, Nephritis, Intestinal colic

HS Basil/*Ocimum basilicum*
HS Ledum/*Rhododendron groenlandicum*
HS Shiso/*Perilla frutescens*
HS Bergamot/*Citrus bergamia*
HS Marjoram/*Origanum majorana*
HS Lavender/*Lavandula vera*
HS Lemon verbena/*Lippia citriodora*

Choose 1–3 of these hydrosols and add 1 tsp. of each to a cup of hot water and drink every 30 minutes based on the situation.

Use hot compresses on the painful zone with the same hydrosols.

Apply locally on the treatment zones essential oils such as ledum, lemon myrtle, lemon basil, lemon petitgrain, shiso or ammi visnaga, every 30 minutes based on the situation.

Hiccups

Add 1 tsp. of basil hydrosol to a cup of water, drink all at once. Repeat after 5 minutes if the symptoms haven't stopped.

Hyperthyroidism (adjuvant)

HS Marjoram/*Origanum majorana*	100 ml
HS Vetiver/*Vetiveria zizanoides*	100 ml

Drink 1 tsp. in a cup of water 3 times a day for 21 days. Stop for 7 days, then restart.

Apply 1 drop of essential oils myrrh and elemi at the base of the neck 3 times a day for 21 days. Stop for 7 days and then restart.

Hypothyroidism (adjuvant)

HS Cinnamon bark/*Cinnamomum verum*	100 ml
HS Myrtle/*Myrtus communis*	100 ml

Drink 1 tsp. in a cup of water 3 times a day for 21 days. Stop for 7 days and then restart.

Apply 1 drop of essential oils myrtle and galangal to the base of the neck for 21 days. Stop for 7 days and then restart.

Indigestion

Choose 1–3 of the hydrosols found in the 'Digestive' section in the therapeutic index. Drink 1–3 tsp. in a cup of hot water, every 30 minutes until the symptoms disappear. Use hot compresses on the stomach.

Infectious diarrhoea (gastroenteritis)

HS Cinnamon/*Cinnamomum verum*	50 ml
HS Savory/*Satureja montana*	25 ml
HS Marjoram/*Origanum majorana*	25 ml
HS Tea tree/*Melaleuca alternifolia*	25 ml
HS Geranium/*Pelargonium asperum*	50 ml

Drink 1 tsp. in a cup of hot water every hour until the symptoms disappear and then continue the treatment for 3–4 days.

Massage the stomach with melaleuca alternifolia and origanum majorana essential oils.

Intestinal fungal infections

HS Tea tree/*Melaleuca alternifolia*	50 ml
HS Geranium/*Pelargonium asperum*	50 ml
HS Palmarosa/*Cymbopogon martini*	50 ml
HS Coriander/*Coriandrum sativum*	50 ml
HS Sandalwood/*Santalum album*	50 ml
HS Cinnamon/*Cinnamomum verum*	50 ml

Drink a cup of hot water with 1 tbsp. of the blend before meals for 40 consecutive days.

For 3 days straight, undertake an intestinal cleansing as an enema with 3 tbsp. of the blend in 1 litre of water or use 3–4 tbsp. of the mix in water for a colonic irrigation.

Liver (congestion)

HS Helichrysum/*Helichrysum italicum*	100 ml
HS Ledum/*Rhododendron groenlandicum*	50 ml
HS Rosemary verbenon/*Rosmarinus verbenoniferum*	50 ml
HS Peppermint/*Mentha piperita*	100 ml

Add 1 tbsp. to 1 litre of hot water to drink during the day for 21 days. Stop for 9 days, then restart if necessary. Ideal after an illness, if you want to break an addiction (alcohol, tobacco, chocolate, etc.) or in case of psoriasis or eczema.

Obesity

It is difficult to suggest a general recipe for reducing weight. Overall food habits are important, and it goes without saying that just drinking a hydrosol will not be enough to reach that body shape you've been dreaming of.

However, hydrosol cures can stimulate the metabolism, have a depurative, diuretic and detoxifying effect, reduce your desire to consume sugar, gluten or lactose, and finally contribute to feeling better about yourself.

Some suggested hydrosols are:

HS Campak/*Michelia alba*: excessive need for sugar, bulimia

HS Sandalwood/*Santalum album*: inability to feel satiety, excessive need for sugar

HS Common juniper/*Juniperus communis*: water retention, excess *kapha*, uric acid, emotional apathy

HS Jasmine/*Jasminum officinalis*: weak digestion and metabolism

HS Savory/*Satureja montana*: slow metabolism, excess *kapha*, weak digestive fire (Agni)

HS Cinnamon bark/*Cinnamomum verum*: introversion, slow metabolism, excess *kapha*

HS Rosemary verbenon/*Rosmarinus ct. verbenoniferum*: progesterone-like, hepatic weakness, metabolic weakness, hepatic and pancreatic failure

HS Scots pine/*Pinus sylvestris*: lymphatic and circulatory stasis, metabolic weakness, excess *kapha*

HS Sage officinalis/*Salvia officinalis*: excessive appetite, excess *pitta* and lack of oestrogen during menopause

HS Everlasting/*Helichrysum italicum*: metabolic weakness, difficulty in overcoming a trauma, excessive appetite

HS Ledum/*Rhododendron groenlandicum*: hepatic, pancreatic and kidney congestion

HS Cypress/*Cupressus sempervirens*: venous and lymphatic stasis, water retention

Choose 3–5 hydrosols and drink 1–2 tbsp. of the blend in 1 litre of hot water during the day for 40 days; restart if necessary.

Vomiting

HS Cinnamon bark/*Cinnamomum verum*

Drink a cup of hot water with 1 tbsp. of this hydrosol each hour until the symptoms stop. If it is not possible to keep down this amount, take half a tsp. every 15 minutes. If the vomiting is linked to motion sickness, use peppermint hydrosol instead. In case of pregnancy, use basil or marjoram hydrosol.

3. Hydrosol therapy for the cardiovascular system

Arrhythmia

Choose from the following hydrosols, personalise the treatment by closely reading the psycho-emotional and energy aspects of the plants.

HS Sandalwood/*Santalum album*
HS Orange blossom/*Citrus aurantium*
HS Kewra/*Pandanus odoratus*
HS Lavender/*Lavandula vera*
HS Marjoram/*Origanum majorana*
HS Spikenard/*Nardostachys jatamansi*
HS Lemon verbena/*Lippia citriodora*
HS Ylang ylang/*Cananga odorata*

Add 1 tbsp. of 1 hydrosol or a mix of hydrosols to 1–1.5 litres of water and drink during the day, or 1 tsp. to a cup of hot water and drink after meals.

Also apply essential oils such as marjoram, lavender, spikenard, neroli, petitgrain bigarade or ylang ylang to the wrists, armpits and solar plexus.

Cellulite

HS Cypress/*Cupressus sempervirens*	50 ml
HS Italian helichrysum/*Helichrysum italicum*	50 ml
HS Common juniper/*Juniperus communis*	50 ml
HS Rosemary verbenon/*Rosmarinus ct. verbenoniferum*	50 ml
HS Sandalwood/*Santalum album*	50 ml
HS Bergamot/*Citrus bergamia*	150 ml

Add 2 tbsp. to 1.5 litres of water and drink during the day for 40 days. Stop for a week, then repeat if necessary.

Spray the affected zone with the same blend before applying massage oil or a natural anti-cellulite cream.

Add 2 tbsp. to bath water.

Suggestions for an anti-cellulite massage oil:

EO Cypress/*Cupressus sempervirens*	1.0 ml
EO Lemon/*Citrus limonum*	2.0 ml
EO Atlas cedar/*Cedrus atlanticum*	0.5 ml
EO Yarrow/*Achillea millefolium*	0.5 ml
EO Sea fennel/*Crithmum maritimum*	0.5 ml
EO Common juniper/*Juniperus communis*	0.5 ml
EO Black spruce/*Picea mariana*	2.0 ml
EO Lemongrass/*Cymbopogon winterianus*	2.0 ml
CO Hazelnut	100.0 ml

Massage the affected zone, morning and evening.

Haematoma

HS Everlasting/*Helichrysum italicum*

Drink 1 tsp. in a cup of water 3–6 times a day until the haematoma disappears.

Externally:

EO Everlasting/*Helichrysum italicum*	2 drops
CO *Calophyllum inophyllum*	4 drops

Massage the haematoma 3–4 times a day with this blend.

Haemorrhoids

HS Yarrow/*Achillea millefolium*	25 ml
HS Spikenard/*Nardostachys jatamansi*	25 ml
HS Cypress/*Cupressus sempervirens*	25 ml
HS Blue camomile/*Chamomilla matricaria*	25 ml
HS Cistus/*Cistus ladaniferus*	25 ml
HS Geranium/*Pelargonium asperum*	75 ml

Drink 1 tbsp. of the mix in 1–1.5 litres of water during the day until the symptoms disappear.

Spray the rectum several times a day with the blend.

Increase the concentration of cistus in cases of bleeding.

Hypertension

Choose among the following hydrosols and personalise the treatment by closely reading the psycho-emotional and energy aspects of the plants.

HS Sandalwood/*Santalum album*
HS Champak/*Michelia alba*
HS Geranium/*Pelargonium asperum*
HS Kewra/*Pandanus odoratum*
HS Lavender/*Lavandula vera*
HS Marjoram/*Origanum majorana*
HS Spikenard/*Nardostachys jatamansi*
HS Rose/*Rosa damascena*
HS Lemon verbena/*Lippia citriodora*
HS Ylang ylang/*Cananga odorata*

Drink 2 tbsp. of a mix of the listed hydrosols or a single one per day. Continue the treatment for 40 days, stop for a week and restart if necessary.

Drinking a cup of hot water before going to bed with Roman camomile and orange blossom hydrosols can also help, as they improve sleep quality.

Also apply essential oils, such as marjoram, lavender, spikenard or ylang ylang, to the wrists, armpits and solar plexus.

Raynaud's disease

HS Cinnamon/*Cinnamomum verum*
HS Cypress/*Cupressus sempervirens*
HS Vetiver/*Vetiveria zizanoides*

Add 1 tsp. of each to 1 litre of hot water and drink during the day starting in the morning for a period of 40 days. Stop for a week and then restart.

Take hot hand baths with 1 tsp. of these hydrosols.

Varicose veins

Choose 3–5 hydrosols from the following list and personalise the treatment by closely reading the psycho-emotional and energy aspects of the plants.

HS Yarrow/*Achillea millefolium*
HS Sandalwood/*Santalum album*
HS Blue camomile/*Camomilla matricaria*
HS Atlas cedar/*Cedrus atlanticum*
HS Cypress/*Cupressus sempervirens*
HS Frankincense/*Boswellia carterii*
HS Geranium/*Pelargonium asperum*
HS Kewra/*Pandanus odoratus*
HS Marjoram/*Origanum majorana*
HS Spikenard/*Nardostachys jatamansi*
HS Myrtle/*Myrtus communis*
HS Scots pine/*Pinus sylvestris*
HS Rose/*Rosa damascena*
HS Vetiver/*Vetiveria zizanoides*

Add 1 tbsp. of the mix to 1.5 litres of hot water and drink during the day for several months.

Externally:
Soak a cotton ball with the hydrosol mix and apply it to the varicose veins for 10–15 minutes a day.

You can also blend some essential oils and apply them twice a day until the symptoms disappear:

EO Mastic tree/*Pistacia lentiscus*	3 drops
EO Cypress/*Cupressus sempervirens*	10 drops
EO Everlasting/*Helichrysum italicum*	3 drops
EO Peppermint/*Mentha piperita*	5 drops
EO Spikenard/*Nardostachys jatamansi*	5 drops
CO *Calophyllum inophyllum* QS	10 ml

Water retention, lymphatic oedema

HS Cypress/*Cupressus sempervirens*
HS Common juniper/*Juniper communis*
HS Helichrysum/*Helichrysum italicum*

Add 1 tbsp. of each to 1.5 litres of water and drink during the day.

4. Hydrosol therapy for the mouth

Buccal hygiene

Mouthwash after brushing with equal parts of bay laurel and tea tree hydrosol.

For sores, spray the lesions with bay laurel and ravintsara hydrosols.

Gargle and rinse the mouth with rose, coriander and peppermint hydrosols in case of bad breath.

Spray the gums or mouthwash with cistus hydrosol in case of bleeding.

Dental abscesses and pain

HS Cinnamon bark/*Cinnamomum verum*	50 ml
HS Savory/*Satureja montana*	50 ml
HS Bay laurel/*Laurus nobilis*	50 ml
HS Peppermint/*Mentha piperita*	50 ml

Spray the mouth cavity and abscess several times a day.

Additionally:

EO Clove/*Eugenia caryophyllata*	1 drop
EO Bay laurel/*Laurus nobilis*	1 drop
EO Peppermint/*Mentha piperita*	1 drop
CO *Rosa rubiginosa*	3 drops

Apply on the abscess 3–5 times a day based on the situation.

Dental extraction

Mouthwash with everlasting and yarrow hydrosols. Spray with cistus hydrosol if there is bleeding. Geranium hydrosol can also be used.

Fever blister/Labial herpes

HS Peppermint
HS Damascus rose

Add 1 tbsp. of each to 1.5 litres of water and drink during the day.

Spray the lesion several times with a blend of these hydrosols or one or the other.

A prolonged 40-day cure will lower the *pitta* bioenergy (irritability, annoyance, gastric acidity, excessive perspiration, redness).

The essential oil of tea tree or peppermint can also be applied to the blisters.

Gingivitis

Mouthwash and spray the gums with bay laurel, peppermint, cinnamon and yarrow hydrosols.

5. Hydrosol therapy for women

Amenorrhoea

HS Sage officinalis/*Salvia officinalis*	50 ml
HS Clary sage/*Salvia sclarea*	70 ml
HS Geranium/*Pelargonium asperum*	50 ml
HS Yarrow/*Achillea millefolium*	30 ml

Add 1 tsp. of the mix to a cup of hot water before meals and drink daily, based on the situation.

Use hot compresses on the stomach in case of cramps.

Add 1–3 tbsp. to bath water.

Massage oil for the stomach and lower back:

EO Clary sage/*Salvia sclarea*	0.5 ml
EO Vetiver/*Vetiveria zizanoides*	0.1 ml
EO Yarrow/*Achillea millefolium*	0.1 ml
EO Sweet fennel/*Foeniculum vulgaris*	0.25 ml
EO Geranium/*Pelargonium asperum*	0.5 ml
CO Hazelnut	15.0 ml
CO Borage QS	30 ml

Massage the stomach and lower back daily.

Childbirth (easing of delivery)

The following remedies are uterotonic and aim to stimulate contractions to ease delivery.

Internally:
Drink daily, 1 week before term; continue if term is exceeded.
1 tbsp. Cinnamon bark hydrosol in 1 litre of water.

Externally:

EO Palmarosa/*Cymbopogon martinii*	1.5 ml
EO Mandarin/*Citrus reticulata leaves*	1.0 ml
EO Clove/*Sizygium aromaticum*	0.5 ml
CO Hazelnut QS	30 ml

Massage the stomach and lower back 2–3 times a day. Start 4 days before term and continue if exceeded. During childbirth, apply every 30 minutes.

Cracked nipples during breastfeeding

HS Lavender/*Lavandula angustifolia*
HS Rose/*Rosa damascena*

Directly spray the nipples several times a day based on need. This is a perfect treatment for breastfeeding mothers.

Decreased libido

HS Sandalwood/*Santalum album*
HS Cinnamon bark/*Cinnamomum verum*
HS Champaca/*Michelia alba*
HS Ylang ylang/*Cananga odorata*

Create a mix with these hydrosols or use them individually in water, as a body splash, auric and air spray and also as an aphrodisiac and exhilarating drink (diluted in water).

Dysmenorrhoea/Painful menstruation

Internally:

HS Yarrow/*Achillea millefolium*	50 ml
HS Basil/*Ocimum basilicum*	100 ml
HS Marjoram/*Origanum majorana*	50 ml
HS Lemon verbena/*Lippia citriodora*	100 ml
HS Clary sage/*Salvia sclarea*	100 ml

Drink 1 tsp. of the mix in a cup of hot water morning and evening. Start about 10 days before menstruation and continue for the first 3 days of the period. Continue the following month and for at least 3 cycles and until the symptoms disappear.

In case of cramps, using hot compresses with the blend on the stomach can also soothe.

EO Yarrow/*Achillea millefolium*	1.0 ml
EO Blue camomile/*Chamomilla matricaria*	1.0 ml
EO Clary sage/*Salvia sclarea*	2.0 ml
CO Hazelnut QS	30 ml

Massage the stomach and lower back in case of pain and cramps.

Endometriosis (adjuvant)

HS Cistus/*Cistus ladaniferus*	200 ml
HS Yarrow/*Achillea millefolium*	100 ml

HS Angelica/*Angelica archangelica*	100 ml
HS Geranium/*Pelargonium asperum*	200 ml

Add 1–2 tbsp. to 1 litre of hot water to drink during the day for a minimum of 6 cycles.

Take regular sitz baths with 1–3 tbsp. of the mix.

Genital herpes

HS Peppermint/*Mentha piperita*	100 ml
HS Rose/*Rosa damascene*	100 ml

Spray the genital zone several times a day with this blend.
Drink 1 litre of water with 1 tbsp. of each hydrosol during the day for 15 days.

Genital itching

Choose among the following hydrosols for genital care:

HS Rose/*Rosa damascena*
HS Tea tree/*Melaleuca alternifolia*
HS Geranium /*Pelargonium asperum*
HS Palmarosa/*Cymbopogon martini*

You can use these hydrosols (as a blend or single) as a daily wash to preserve the health and moistness of the vaginal flora.

A sitz bath with these hydrosols can also refresh and bring relief.

You can also spray regularly the itching area (internally and externally).

Hot flashes

HS Sage officinalis/*Salvia officinalis*	50 ml
HS Peppermint/*Mentha piperita*	50 ml
HS Rose/*Rosa damascena*	100 ml
HS Vitex/*Agnus castus*	50 ml

Add 1–2 tbsp. to 1–1.5 litres of water and drink during the day based on the situation.

Regularly spray the face and body with rose hydrosol.

Menopause

Menopause symptoms can manifest themselves in very different ways for each woman. It is advised to make a 50 ml mix with a minimum of 3 hydrosols based on the specific needs of each person (a blend of hydrosols is more effective than using them individually).

HS Clary sage/*Salvia sclarea*: mood swings, low morale and hot flashes, oestrogen-like

HS Yarrow/*Achillea millefolium*: hormonal balancer, builds confidence, ideal for transitional periods

HS Sage officinalis/*Salvia officinalis*: oestrogen-like, rushes on food and hot flashes

HS Cypress/*Cupressus sempervirens*: hormonal balancer, psycho-emotional balancer, diuretic, vasoconstrictor

HS Geranium/*Pelargonium asperum*: anxiolytic, anti-depressant, nervous regulator

HS Kewra/*Pandanus odoratus*: cardiovascular regulator, metabolic stimulant, depurative

HS Peppermint/*Mentha piperita*: supports mental clarity, soothes *pitta* and hot flashes

HS Rose/*Rosa damascena*: balances irritability and hot flashes

HS Carrot/*Daucus carota*: for urogenital tract and liver regeneration, for its depurative properties, supports confidence

HS Rosemary verbenon/*Rosmarinus verbenoniferum*: depurative, metabolic and hepatic stimulant and progesterone-like

HS Vitex/*Agnus castus*: metabolic stimulant, progesterone-like, works on hot flashes

Drink 1 tbsp. of the mix in 1 litre of hot water during the day. Continue the treatment for several months if necessary.

Menorrhagia

Internally:

HS Cistus/*Cistus ladaniferus*	200 ml
and/or	
HS Yarrow/*Achillea millefolium*	200 ml

Add 1 tbsp. of the mix (equal parts) or 1 tsp. of each hydrosol to 1 litre of hot water to drink during the day. Start 1 week before periods and continue to drink throughout the menstruation. Restart every month until the cycle is harmonised and until periods are less abundant.

Nausea during pregnancy

Internally:

HS Bergamot/*Citrus bergamia*	100 ml
HS Basil/*Ocimum basilicum*	100 ml
HS Orange blossom/*Citrus aurantium*	100 ml

In cases of severe morning sickness, take 1 tsp. of the mix 3 times a day before meals. If necessary, take an additional 1 tsp. before getting up.

Premature contractions

Drink 1 litre of water with 3 tbsp. of kewra hydrosol during the day. Use a compress soaked with this hydrosol on the stomach. Massage the lower back with relaxing massage oil, for example:

EO Lavender/*Lavandula angustifolia*	2.0 ml
EO Petitgrain bigarade/*Citrus aurantifolium* (leaves)	3.0 ml
EO Neroli/*Citrus aurantifolium* (flowers)	0.2 ml
CO Hazelnut	100.0 ml

Premenstrual syndrome

Premenstrual syndrome can manifest itself in varied ways based on each woman. Create a blend with a minimum of 3 hydrosols based on specific needs. A blend of hydrosols is more effective than using them individually.

Internally:

HS Yarrow/*Achillea millefolium*: lack of confidence, psycho-emotional imbalance, hormonal imbalance

HS Geranium/*Pelargonium asperum*: hormonal and psycho-emotional imbalance, depression

HS Clary sage/*Salvia sclarea*: hormonal imbalance, fear, anxiety, psycho-emotional imbalance, excessive appetite, cramps

HS Lemon verbena/*Lippia citriodora*: cramps, nervousness, psycho-emotional imbalance, depression

HS Vitex/*Agnus castus*: metabolic imbalances, lack of progesterone, hot flashes

HS Rose/*Rosa damascena*: hot flashes and irritability

HS Cypress/*Cupressus sempervirens*: lack of emotional control, water retention

HS Juniper/*Juniperus communis*: fatigue and water retention

HS Basil/*Ocimum basilicum*: swollen abdomen

HS St John's wort/*Hypericum perforatum*: depression and insomnia

HS Sandalwood/*Santalum album*: mental agitation and constipation

Choose 50 ml of 3 hydrosols and take 1 tbsp. of the blend in 1 litre of hot water to drink during the day: start 1 week before period and continue throughout the cycle.

Restart each month until symptoms disappear.

Urogenital tract inflammations and infections

HS Cinnamon/*Cinnamomum verum*	75 ml
HS Sandalwood/*Santalum album*	75 ml
HS Thyme linalool/*Thymus vulgaris linaloliferum*	75 ml

Add 6 tbsp. in 2 litres of water to drink during the day (for 21 days).

Uterine fibroids (adjuvant)

HS Cistus/*Cistus ladaniferus*	50 ml
HS Cypress/*Cupressus sempervirens*	50 ml
HS Yarrow/*Achillea millefolium*	50 ml
HS Shiso/*Perilla frutescens*	50 ml

HS Angelica/*Angelica archangelica*	50 ml
HS Geranium/*Pelargonium asperum*	100 ml
HS Ylang ylang/*Cananga odorata*	100 ml

Add 1–2 tbsp. to 1 litre of hot water to drink during the day for 4 months.

Regularly take sitz baths with 1–3 tbsp. of the blend.

Increase the cistus hydrosols concentration in case of haemorrhagic periods.

Vaginal fungal infections

HS Tea tree/*Melaleuca alternifolia*	50 ml
HS Geranium/*Pelargonium asperum*	100 ml
HS Thyme linalool/*Thymus vulgaris linaloliferum*	100 ml
HS Vetiver/*Vetiveria zizanoides*	50 ml
HS Bergamot/*Citrus bergamia*	100 ml

Use vaginal douches mixed with $^1/_2$ water and $^1/_2$ hydrosol blend.

Regularly spray the intimate zone.

For 40 days, drink 1 litre of water with 1–2 tbsp. of the blend a day.

Vaginitis/Vulvitis

HS Tea tree/*Melaleuca alternifolia*	50 ml
HS Rose/*Rosa damascena*	50 ml
HS Sweet thyme/*Thymus vulgaris linaloliferum*	50 ml
HS Cinnamon/*Cinnamomum verum* (not during pregnancy)	30 ml
HS Vetiver/*Vetiveria zizanoides*	30 ml
HS Palmarosa/*Cymbopogon martinii* (not during pregnancy)	50 ml
Water	1 litre

Use a vaginal enema/douche 2–4 times a day using 100 ml of the mix; for the 2 first days, you can also use enemas with undiluted hydrosols. Use compresses soaked with the blend and place on external genital parts.

6. Hydrosol therapy and the urogenital system

Cystitis

Internally:

HS Lemon verbena/*Lippia citriodora*	100 ml
HS Sandalwood/*Santalum album*	50 ml
HS Cinnamon/*Cinnamomum verum*	50 ml
HS Savory/*Satureja montana*	50 ml
HS Marjoram/*Origanum majorana*	50 ml
HS Cypress/*Cupressus sempervirens*	50 ml

Add 1 tsp. of the blend to a cup of hot water and drink 4–6 times a day for 2 weeks.

Use hot compresses soaked with the blend on the lower back.

Use sitz baths with the blend.

You can also use juniper, palmarosa, yarrow, Scots pine, tea tree and kewra hydrosols.

For prevention:
Drink hot water with 1 tsp. of sandalwood or bergamot hydrosol daily to activate the circulation of the pelvic area.

Kidney lithiasis (adjuvant)

Undertake a cure with juniper, lemon verbena and cinnamon hydrosols, 3 tbsp. in total (1 of each or you can vary per day) in 1 litre of water to drink during the day for 21 days. Stop for 7 days, and then restart. Repeat the cycle a minimum of 3 times.

Or:

HS Cinnamon/*Cinnamomum verum*	100 ml
HS Lemon verbena/*Lippia citriodora*	100 ml
HS Kewra/*Pandanus odoratus*	100 ml
HS Juniper/*Juniperus communis*	100 ml

Add 4 tbsp. to 1 litre of hot water and drink during the day. Use compresses soaked with the blend to place on the painful zone. Undertake a 21-day cure, stop for 7 days and then restart a minimum of 3 times. Also take essential oil ammi visnaga internally (2–4 drops a day).

Massage the zone:

EO Common juniper/*Juniperus communis*	2.0 ml
EO Lemongrass/*Cymbopogon flexuosus*	3.0 ml
EO Sea fennel/*Crithmum maritimum*	1.0 ml
EO Basil (ct. methylchavicol)/*Ocimum basilicum*	2.0 ml
EO Katafray/*Cedrelopsis grevei*	2.0 ml
CO *Calophyllum inophyllum*	20 ml
CO St John's wort	50 ml

Prostatitis

Internally:

HS Cypress/*Cupressus sempervirens*	100 ml
HS Scots pine/*Pinus sylvestris*	100 ml
HS Sandalwood/*Santalum album*	100 ml
HS Peppermint/*Mentha piperita*	100 ml

Add 1 tsp. to a cup of hot water and drink in the morning and before lunch for 40 days. Stop for 7 days and then restart if necessary.

Use compresses soaked with the blend to place on the pubis in an attack.

Pyelonephritis (adjuvant)

Internally:

HS Kewra/*Pandanus odoratus*	100 ml
HS Juniper/*Juniperus communis*	100 ml
HS Palmarosa/*Cymbopogon martinii*	100 ml
HS St John's wort/*Hypericum perforatum*	100 ml
HS Bergamot/*Citrus bergamia*	100 ml

HS Scots pine/*Pinus sylvestris*   100 ml

Add 3 tbsp. to 1 litre of hot water and drink during the day.

Use hot compresses soaked with the blend on painful zones.

Renal failure

Undertake a cure choosing 3 hydrosols among the following. Drink 1.5 litres of water with 3 tbsp. of the mix.

HS Yarrow/*Achillea millefolium*
HS Angelica/*Angelica archangelica*
HS Sandalwood/*Santalum album*
HS Atlas cedar/*Cedrus atlanticum*
HS Juniper/*Juniper communis*
HS Scots pine/*Pinus sylvestris*
HS Ledum/*Rhododendron groenlandicum*
HS Vetiver/*Vetiveria zizanoides*

Sexual dysfunction in men

Morning and noon, drink a cup of hot water with 1 tsp. of Scots pine hydrosol.

At night, drink a cup of hot water with 1 tsp. of sandalwood hydrosol.

Spray the stomach and genitals with sandalwood hydrosol.

You can also use champaca, jasmine, kewra, angelica or ylang ylang hydrosols.

Massage the adrenal gland with the essential oils of black spruce or hemlock spruce.

Massage the lower stomach and genitals with the essential oil sandalwood (10% in CO).

Water retention

Internally:

HS Juniper/*Juniperus communis*   100 ml
HS Cypress/*Cupressus sempervirens*   100 ml

| HS Rosemary/*Rosmarinus off. verbenoniferum* | 100 ml |
| HS Scots pine/*Pinus sylvestris* | 100 ml |

Add 1–2 tbsp. to 1 litre of water and drink during the day.

7. Hydrosol therapy for the skin

Acne

Drink 1 litre of water with 1 tbsp. of each hydrosol: rosemary verbenon and ledum.

Make a clay mask by choosing hydrosols such as cistus, coriander, geranium, *helichrysum italicum*, bay laurel, lavender, myrtle, palmarosa, rose or thyme linalool (see the specifics of each).

Use the same hydrosols as a tonic after washing, morning and night.

Aromatherapy:
Apply to each pimple an essential oil or mix, such as spike lavender, tea tree, saro, rosalina or thyme linalool.

Chicken pox

Generously spray the body with ravintsara hydrosol.

Drink a cup of hot water with 1 tsp. of the same hydrosol per day until the symptoms disappear.

Cutaneous abscesses

Internally:

HS Rose/*Rosa damascena*	100 ml
HS Ledum/*Rhododendron groenlandicum*	100 ml
HS Geranium/*Pelargonium asperum*	100 ml
HS Carrot/*Daucus carota*	100 ml

Add 2 tbsp. of the blend to 1 litre of hot water and drink during the day.

Externally:

Regularly spray the blend on the area to treat.

EO Holy basil/*Ocimum basilicum sanctum*	1 drop
EO Tea tree/*Melaleuca alternifolia*	1 drop
EO Saro/*Cinnamosma fragrans*	1 drop
CO *Calophyllum inophyllum*	0.5 ml

Three local applications per day, based on the situation.

Cutaneous allergies

Spray the treatment zone several times a day with blue camomile hydrosol. Also drink 1 litre of water with 2 tbsp. of the hydrosol during the day.

Eczema

Generously spray in case of itching with hydrosols such as yarrow, sandalwood, blue camomile, champaca, coriander, geranium, lavender, peppermint or rose (see specificities of each).

Use compresses with said hydrosols on the affected zone.

Internally:

HS Sandalwood/*Santalum album*	100 ml
HS Myrtle/*Myrtus communis*	100 ml
HS Lavender/*Lavandula angustifolia*	100 ml
HS Shiso/*Perilla frutescens*	100 ml

Add 2 tbsp. to 1.5 litres of water and drink during the day for 40 days.

Eyelids (irritation, infection)

Spray the eyelids several times a day with hydrosols such as Roman camomile, champaca, lavender or myrtle.

Excessive perspiration

For the menopause (see menopause).

Otherwise, internally:

HS Rose/*Rosa damascena*	50 ml
HS Sage/*Salvia officinalis*	50 ml
HS Peppermint/*Mentha piperita*	50 ml
HS Cistus/*Cistus ladaniferus*	50 ml

Energy and/or Ayurvedic properties: diminishes *pitta*

Add 1 tbsp. of the mix to 1.5 litres of hot water and drink during the day based on the situation until symptoms disappear.

Fungal infections: skin and nails

HS Tea tree/*Melaleuca alternifolia*	50 ml
HS Thyme linalool/*Thymus vulgaris linaloliferum*	50 ml
HS Vetiver/*Vetiveria zizanoides*	50 ml
HS Geranium/*Pelargonium asperum*	100 ml

Spray the affected area 3–4 times a day; also drink 1 tsp. in a cup of hot water 3 times a day.

Aromatherapy:

EO Ahibero/*Cymbopogon giganteus*	3.0 ml
EO Rose geranium/*Pelargonium asperum*	3.0 ml
EO Manuka/*Leptospermum scoparium*	0.5 ml
EO Palmarosa/*Cymbopogon martinii*	3.0 ml
EO Cinnamon bark/*Cinnamomum verum*	0.5 ml
CO *Argan* QS	30 ml

Apply locally on the mycosis (5–8 drops) 2–5 times a day based on the situation.

General skincare

Hydrosols are often excellent tonics and can be used morning and night after skin cleaning and before applying a facial cream. However, it is important to use only 100 per cent vegetal and natural products if you include essential oils and hydrosols. Here are some suggestions:

HS Sandalwood/*Santalum album*: dry skin, acne, irritated and sensitive skin, itching

HS Blue camomile/*Camomilla matricaria*: hypersensitive and reactive skin, rosacea, irritated skin

HS Carrot/*Daucus carota*: tired and degenerated skin, rosacea

HS Cistus/*Cistus ladaniferus*: acne, weak microcirculation of the skin

HS Cypress/*Cupressus sempervirens*: acne, eczema, rosacea

HS Frankincense/*Boswellia carterii*: mature skin, wrinkles

HS Eucalyptus/*Eucalyptus globulus*: oily skin, acne

HS Orange blossom/*Citrus aurantium*: all skin types

HS Geranium/*Pelargonium asperum*: acne, razor burn, wounds/cuts

HS Everlasting/*Helichrysum italicum*: acne, scars, rosacea, redness

HS Lavender/*Lavandula vera*: irritated and sensitive skin

HS Peppermint/*Mentha piperita*: weak microcirculation of the skin, sunburn, acne

HS Myrtle/*Myrtus communis*: acne, rosacea, dull skin

HS Spikenard/*Nardostachys jatamansi*: psoriasis, eczema, mature skin, wrinkles

HS Palmarosa/*Cymbopogon martinii*: acne, razor burn, combination skin

HS Rose/*Rosa damascena*: dull, mature and combination skin

HS Scots pine/*Pinus sylvestris*: grey and weak microcirculation of the skin, smokers

HS Clary sage/*Salvia sclarea*: dull and tired skin

HS Thyme linalool/*Thymus vulgaris linaloliferum*: acne, eczema, sensitive skin

HS Vetiver/*Vetiveria zizanoides*: tired, dry and irritated skin, rosacea, *vata* skin

Hives

HS Peppermint/*Mentha piperita*	50 ml
HS Ylang ylang/*Cananga odorata*	50 ml
HS Coriander/*Coriandrum sativum*	50 ml
HS Rose/*Rosa damascena*	50 ml
HS Blue camomile/*Camomilla matricaria*	50 ml

As a spray:
Spray the treatment zone several times a day until the symptoms disappear.

Use a 'liver decongestion' treatment at the same time.

Loss of hair

According to Ayurveda, hair loss is often linked to excess *pitta* and hepatic congestion. You can make a mix of 3 hydrosols from the following list based on personal needs:

HS Lavender/*Lavandula vera* and/or Peppermint/*Mentha piperita*: if you often sweat and have an itchy scalp

HS Atlas cedar/*Cedrus atlantica* and/or Spikenard/*Nardostachys jatamansi*: lack of vitality of hair, fine hair and in case of scalp psoriasis

HS Sage/*Salvia officinalis*: hair loss during menopause

HS Rosemary verbenon/*Rosmarinus off. Ct. verbenoniferum* and/or Cypress/*Cupressus sempervirens*: dandruff and oily hair

HS Scots pine/*Pinus sylvestris* and/or Myrtle/*Myrtus communis*: for those who smoke or have a congested lymphatic system

HS Bay laurel/*Laurus nobilis*: feelings of discouragement, thoughts that nothing is going as it should

HS Tea tree/*Melaleuca alternifolia*, Thyme linalool/*Thymus vulgaris linaloliferum* and Vetiver/*Vetiveria zizanoides*: scalp mycosis

Spray the scalp with the chosen blend after shampooing, and vigorously massage it twice a day based on the situation. Add to the last rinse after shampooing.

Internally:
Drink 1 tbsp. of the mix in 1.5 litres of water during the day for 40 days. Stop for 40 days, then restart.

Pruritus

HS Blue camomile/*Chamomilla matricaria*	50 ml
HS Lavender/*Lavandula angustifolia*	50 ml
HS Peppermint/*Mentha piperita*	50 ml
HS Everlasting/*Helichrysum italicum*	50 ml

Spray the affected zone several times a day until symptoms disappear.

Psoriasis

HS Spikenard/*Nardostachys jatamansi*	50 ml

HS Geranium/*Pelargonium asperum*	100 ml
HS Atlas cedar/*Cedrus atlanticum*	50 ml
HS Blue camomile/*Chamomilla matricaria*	50 ml
HS Everlasting/*Helichrysum italicum*	50 ml

Spray the affected zone 2–3 times a day.

Internally:
Take the 'liver (congestion)' mix internally.

Rosacea

HS Cypress/*Cupressus sempervirens*	50 ml
HS Helichrysum/*Helichrysum italicum*	50 ml
HS Peppermint/*Mentha piperita*	50 ml
HS Coriander/*Coriandrum sativum*	50 ml

Use as a tonic morning and night after cleaning the face and before applying an appropriate natural cream.

Undertake a hydrosol cure internally (see varicose veins).

Shingles

HS Peppermint/*Mentha piperita*	100 ml
HS Ravintsara/*Cinnamomum camphora*	100 ml
HS Rose/*Rosa damascena*	100 ml

Add 2 tbsp. of the blend to 1.5 litres of hot water and drink during the day for 40 days; restart if necessary.

Spray or use compresses on the affected zone with the same blend.

Aromatherapy:

EO Peppermint/*Mentha piperita*	3.5 ml
EO Ravintsara/*Cinnamomum camphora*	3.5 ml
CO *Calophyllum inophyllum* QS	20.0 ml

Apply a couple of drops of the mix to the affected zone several times a day.

Sunburn

Spray the affected zone with lavender and/or rose and/or everlasting hydrosols.

8. Hydrosol therapy for the psycho-emotional system

Addictions (tobacco, alcohol, drugs, etc.)

HS Bergamot/*Citrus bergamia*	50 ml
HS Orange blossom/*Citrus aurantium*	50 ml
HS Myrtle/*Myrtus communis*	50 ml
HS Champak/*Michelia alba*	50 ml

Spray the mouth and around the body when faced with a craving. Add 2 tbsp. of the mix to 1 litre of water and drink during the day, based on the situation.

Aggressiveness and angry attitude

In this case, it is important to reduce the *pitta* fire bioenergy. Choose from the following hydrosols based on their specifics. It is also useful to use plants that regenerate the liver, such as ledum.

HS Yarrow/*Achillea millefolium*: difficulty accepting change, unable to understand the opposite sex

HS Sandalwood/*Santalum album*: Cartesian mind, perfection, dissatisfaction

HS Blue camomile/*Chamomilla matricaria*: self-judgement, dissatisfaction, unable to see the big picture

HS Champaca/*Michelia alba*: unable to feel love

HS Coriander/*Coriandrum sativum*: explosive temperament, short fuse, can't see reality for what it is

HS Frankincense/*Boswellia carterii*: rigid mind, Cartesian mind, lack of spiritual openness

HS Orange blossom/*Citrus aurantium*: fears, phobias

HS Kewra/*Pandanus odoratus*: anger combined with an oppressed heart

HS Marjoram/*Origanum majorana*: projection of false realities

HS St John's wort/*Hypericum perforatum*: fears, anxiety, projections

HS Spikenard/*Nardostachys jatamansi*: unable to focus, to relativise

HS Palmarosa/*Cymbopogon martini*: guilt makes you angry

HS Rose/*Rosa damascena*: resentment, unable to love

HS Clary sage/*Salvia sclarea*: anger brought on by hormonal problems

HS Lemon verbena/*Lippia citriodora*: stuck in a situation, difficulty in turning the page

Undertake a 40-day cure with 1–2 tbsp. in 1 litre of water to drink during the day.

Use the hydrosols as an auric and ambiance spray, in the bath or add to a face mask.

Anorexia

HS Bergamot/*Citrus bergamia*	100 ml
HS Lemon verbena/*Lippia citriodora*	100 ml
HS Cinnamon/*Cinnamomum verum*	100 ml

Add 2 tbsp. to 1 litre of water and drink during the day. Use the blend as an auric and air spray.

Anxiety (after mourning)

Add 1 tsp. of lemon verbena hydrosol to a cup of hot water and drink 3–5 times a day based on the situation. Also use this hydrosol as an auric and air spray.

Anxiety (fear of the unknown)

Add 1 tsp. of vetiver hydrosol and 1 tsp. of orange blossom hydrosol to a cup of hot water and drink 3–5 times a day based on the situation.

You can also use Roman camomile, blue camomile, St John's wort or spikenard hydrosols.

Apathy, indifference with regards to relationships

HS Jasmine/*Jasminum officinalis*	100 ml
HS Kewra/*Pandanus odoratus*	50 ml
HS Scots pine/*Pinus sylvestris*	100 ml

Add 2 tbsp. to 1 litre of water and drink during the day. Use the blend as an auric and air spray.

Insomnia

Insomnia can manifest itself in many ways based on the individual. It is advised to make a 200 ml blend with a minimum of 3 hydrosols based on specific needs.

HS Yarrow/*Achillea millefolium*: unable to accept change
HS Roman camomile/*Chamaemelum nobilis*: fear, anxiety, unable to let go
HS Vetiver/*Vetiveria zizanoides*: agitation, fear, hypertension
HS Orange blossom/*Citrus aurantium*: concern, fear, anxiety
HS St John's wort/*Hypericum perforatum*: depression, anxiety, fear
HS Lemon verbena/*Lippia citriodora*: unable to turn the page, stuck in a rut
HS Lavender/*Lavandula vera*: mental rigidity, perfectionist mind
HS Marjoram/*Origanum majorana*: hypertension, anxiety
HS Ravintsara/*Cinnamomum camphora*: lack of clarity, confusion

Add 1 tsp. of the mix to a cup of hot water and drink before bed.

Memory (weakness)

HS Rosemary/*Rosmarinus verbenoniferum*	50 ml
HS Ledum/*Rhododendron groenlandicum*	50 ml
HS Shiso/*Perilla frutescens*	50 ml
HS Coriander/*Coriandrum sativum*	150 ml

Add 1 tbsp. of the blend to 1 litre of hot water and drink during the day.

Mental agitation, nervousness, scatter-brain, difficulty remaining focused and concentrated

In this case, it is important to reduce the *vata* (air) bioenergy and undertake a cure with a blend that builds confidence and calms the mind. Choose hydrosols that come from roots or wood, such as sandalwood, carrot, atlas cedar, spikenard or vetiver. Combine with other calming hydrosols such as orange blossom, Roman camomile or marjoram.

For example:

HS Vetiver/*Vetiveria zizanoides*	50 ml
HS Orange blossom/*Citrus aurantium*	100 ml
HS Basil/*Ocimum basilicum*	50 ml
HS Roman camomile/*Chamaemelum nobile*	50 ml

Drink a cup of hot water with 1 tsp. of the mix 3 times a day.

Add to bath water (3 tbsp.).

Use the mix as an auric or air spray.

Nervous breakdown

HS St John's wort/*Hypericum perforatum*	50 ml
HS Orange blossom/*Citrus aurantium*	50 ml
HS Marjoram/*Origanum majorana*	50 ml
HS Scots pine/*Pinus sylvestris*	50 ml

Add 1 tsp. of the blend to a glass of hot water and drink morning and night (also see section on stress).

Shock

| HS Angelica/*Angelica archangelica* | 50 ml |
| HS Orange blossom/*Citrus aurantium* | 50 ml |

Add 1 tsp. to a cup of water and drink 3–5 times a day, based on the situation.

Use the blend as an auric and air spray.

Sorrow

HS Angelica/*Angelica archangelica*	50 ml
HS Lemon verbena/*Lippia citriodora*	50 ml
HS Champak/*Michelia alba*	50 ml
HS Rose/*Rosa damascena*	50 ml

Add 2 tbsp. to 1 litre of water and drink during the day. Use the blend as an auric and air spray.

Stress

The causes that bring on stress are multiple, and its manifestation as well. Mix 3 hydrosols that best fit the specific needs.

HS Yarrow/*Achillea millefolium*: caught up by events

HS Angelica/*Angelica archangelica*: difficulty in making decisions

HS Basil/*Ocimum basilicum*: brain is scattered and drowning in emotions

HS Sandalwood/*Santalum album*: having high expectations of life

HS Blue camomile/*Chamomilla matricaria*: perfectionist mind

HS Roman camomile/*Chamaemelum nobilis*: the smallest thing bothers you

HS Carrot/*Daucus carota*: lack of confidence, fear of loss

HS Atlas cedar/*Cedrus atlantica*: others often decide for you

HS Coriander/*Coriandrum sativum*: lack of clarity

HS Frankincense/*Boswellia carterii*: mental rigidity

HS Orange blossom/*Citrus aurantium*: anxiety, fear

HS Kewra/*Pandanus odoratus*: oppressed heart and respiration

HS Lavender/*Lavandula vera*: too attached to mental plans

HS Bay laurel/*Laurus nobilis*: lacking courage to tell the truth

HS Marjoram/*Origanum majorana*: difficulty in living in the present, frayed nerves

HS Clary sage/*Salvia sclarea*: fear of risk, lack of creativity or ideas

HS Spikenard/*Nardostachys jatamansi*: lack of certainty, feeling apathetic, annoyed

HS Rose/*Rosa damascena*: stressed by affective links, feeling imprisoned

HS Lemon verbena/*Lippia citriodora*: unable to turn the page

Add 1 tbsp. to 1.5 litres of water and drink during the day for 40 days.

9. Hydrosol therapy for babies and young children

* *Difficulty sleeping, nightmares:* orange blossom hydrosol in the bottle (1 tsp.), spray the blanket, add 1 tbsp. to bath water.

* *Baby cries a lot, complains, colic, difficult digestion:* Roman camomile hydrosol in the bottle (1 tsp.), add 1 tbsp. in the bath, breastfeeding mother can take it internally, spray nipples with it before breastfeeding, massage the baby's stomach with 1 tbsp. of carrier oil and 3 drops of the same essential oil.

- *Cutaneous problems, allergies:* Blue camomile hydrosol sprayed on affected zones, add 1 tbsp. to the bath water.

- *Teething:* massage the gums with Roman camomile essential oil, spray the gums with Roman camomile hydrosol.

- *To ease the move out of the crib:* rose and orange blossom hydrosol, used as an auric spray, and also spray the mouth before moving.

- *Dysentery/diarrhoea:* hot compresses of tea tree and marjoram hydrosols, after massaging the stomach clockwise with 2 tbsp. of macadamia or another carrier oil and 2 drops of each tea tree and marjoram essential oils. Spray the mouth with the 2 hydrosols several times a day.

- *Chicken pox:* spray the lesions with equal parts of ravintsara and peppermint hydrosols for the virucidal effect and to calm itching.

- *Measles:* $1/3$ peppermint, $1/3$ ravintsara, $1/3$ rose hydrosols taken internally and sprayed on the body.

- Spray the child *who is 'temperamental', who rages,* with Roman camomile or rose hydrosol.

- *Sores, thrush:* spray the mouth with bay laurel hydrosol, alternating with ravintsara hydrosol.

- *Cracked nipples:* spray with cistus hydrosol.

- Wash child's feet if they have *plantar warts* with tea tree hydrosol.

- *Baby's eyes stuck closed on awakening:* Roman camomile and rose hydrosols.

- *Constipation:* spray lemon verbena or bergamot hydrosol in the mouth. Also, 1 tsp. of the same hydrosols in apple juice is soothing.

- *Nappy rash:* spray the bottom with geranium, Roman camomile, rose or thyme linalol hydrosols.

- *Sore throat:* for chidren under 5, spray the throat with rose and/or coriander hydrosols.

- *Cold/rhinitis:* use myrtle and thyme linalool hydrosol as a nasal spray, in the bath and also as an air spray.

* *Lack of appetite:* spray the mouth with bergamot hydrosol or add 1 tsp. to the bottle.

* *Bed-wetting:* blend cypress and marjoram hydrosols in equal parts. Drink 3 times a day a glass of water with 10 drops of the mix before meals until the symptoms disappear. Also blend 1 ml of cypress essential oil with 9 ml of CO and massage the lower stomach 1 hour before sleep.

* *Fever:* use compresses around the feet and spray the body with lavender hydrosol.

10. Hydrosol therapy for rheumatism and osteoarticular problems

For rheumatism, generally it is enough to undertake depurative cures 2–3 times a year to soothe the pain and detoxify the body. Make a blend choosing from among the following hydrosols (see their specifics):

HS Yarrow/*Achillea millefolium*: anti-inflammatory, circulatory tonic, calming

HS Angelica/*Angelica archangelica*: anti-inflammatory, spasmolytic, analgesic, hepatic, pancreatic and metabolic stimulant

HS Bergamot/*Citrus bergamia*: anti-inflammatory, analgesic, hepatic, pancreatic and metabolic stimulant

HS Sandalwood/*Santalum album*: anti-inflammatory, analgesic, diuretic

HS Blue camomile/*Camomilla matricaria*: analgesic and anti-inflammatory, calming

HS Cinnamon bark/*Cinnamomum verum*: anti-inflammatory and analgesic, metabolic, hepatic and pancreatic stimulant

HS Carrot/*Daucus carota*: depurative and regenerative for the gallbladder and kidneys, blood purifier

HS Atlas cedar/*Cedrus atlantica*: depurative, anti-parasitic, litholytic

HS Cypress/*Cupressus sempervirens*: stimulates pancreatic, hepatic and kidney functions

HS Frankincense/*Boswellia carterii*: analgesic and anti-inflammatory

HS Common juniper/*Juniperus communis*: diuretic and anti-inflammatory, hepatic, kidney and pancreatic stimulant, depurative

HS Kewra/*Pandanus odoratus*: analgesic, anti-inflammatory, hepatic and pancreatic depurative

HS Ledum/*Rhododendron groenlandicum*: depurative, detoxifying, hepatic, pancreatic and kidney regenerator, metabolic stimulant

HS Marjoram/*Origanum majorana*: analgesic, decongestant, anti-inflammatory

HS St John's wort/*Hypericum perforatum*: anti-inflammatory, analgesic, calming

HS Scots pine/*Pinus sylvestris*: depurative, draining, diuretic, analgesic, anti-inflammatory, decongestant

HS Rosemary verbenon/*Rosmarinus ct. verbenoniferum*: hepatic, gallbladder and pancreatic regenerator, metabolic stimulant, depurative

HS Shiso/*Perilla frutescens*: depurative and detoxifying, powerful anti-inflammatory and analgesic, hepatic, gallbladder and pancreatic stimulant

Create a blend with 3–6 different hydrosols. Undertake 40-day cures 3 times a year with 2 tbsp. of the blend added to 1 litre of hot water and drunk during the day.

Also use the blend as a hot compress on painful areas.

Add to bath water with alkalising salt (Himalaya salt, for example).

Scrub with Himalaya salt and a St John's wort oil on painful area. (Mix a handful of salt with 1–2 tbsp. of carrier oil and 1–2 tbsp. of the blend, rub the affected area.)

11. Hydrosol therapy for various problems

Care for your feet

* Use foot baths with palmarosa and sage officinalis hydrosols in case of malodorous and excessive perspiration. Also use the 2 hydrosols to regularly spray the feet.

* Spray swollen feet with peppermint and cedar hydrosols or use a foot bath with these hydrosols.

Cold extremities

HS Everlasting/*Helichrysum italicum*	100 ml
HS Cinnamon/*Cinnamomum verum*	100 ml

Add 1 tbsp. to 1 litre of hot water and drink during the day. Massage the extremities with essential oil of ginger blended with a carrier oil (10% concentration).

Eye care

- Compresses with rose hydrosol in cases of inflammation.

- Regularly spray the eyes with rose hydrosol when working in front of a screen.

- Spray irritated eyes or use compresses with myrtle and/or blue camomile hydrosol for allergies.

- For styes, apply compresses with myrtle hydrosol.

- For swollen eyelids, apply compresses with myrtle hydrosol.

- In the case of shingles of the eyes, apply compresses with ravintsara and myrtle hydrosols (equal parts).

Fever

Spray the body with lavender, coriander and/or rose hydrosol. Drink 1 litre of hot water with 1 tbsp. of each hydrosol during the day until symptoms disappear.

Headaches

HS Peppermint/*Mentha piperita*	100 ml
HS Coriander/*Coriandrum sativum*	100 ml

Add 1 tsp. to 1 glass of water and drink every 30 minutes until the symptoms disappear.

Use cold compresses soaked with the blend on the forehead. Apply a drop of peppermint essential oil on the forehead, temples and cervical area.

Neuralgia, chronic headaches

Drink 1 litre of hot water with 2 tbsp. of yarrow hydrosol during the day and apply compresses with this hydrosol.

Glossary of Ayurvedic Terms

AGNI: biological fire that regulates metabolism, cosmic force, transmutation. In Hinduism and Buddhism, Agni is also revered as the god of fire. He is a purifier and destroyer of evil and thus allows regeneration. He is the main witness in the Hindu marriage, the one who ensures the passion of the couple, which allows the cooking of food as well as the transformation of suffering into happiness.

AHAMKARA: ego, a part of the intellect. *Aham* is the self or 'I' and *kara* is 'any created thing' or 'to do'.

AJNA: the 6th chakra, the third eye, located between the eyebrows. It's associated with light and the need to contribute.

AMA: toxins, food that is not digested, or food that has not been eliminated. Literally *ama* means not cooked or not digested. In the Ayurvedic concept, *ama* represents everything that has not been completely transformed, such as food, but also thoughts, emotions and all sensory impressions.

ANAHATA: the heart chakra, located in the centre of the chest. It is associated with the air element and the need for love.

BUDDHI: intelligence freed from the perceptions of the intellect and the ego.

DHARMA: destiny, laws, mission, the path.

DHATUS: the 7 vital tissues of the body.

DOSHAS: the 3 subtle energies, called *vata*, *pitta* and *kapha*.

GUNA: the 3 fundamental attributes as *sattva*, *rajas* and *tamas*.

KAPHA: the bioenergy composed by water and earth element, the subtle energy of *kapha*.

KARMA: causes and consequences. Every act (*karma*) induces effects, supposed to affect the different lives of an individual and create a part of destiny.

MANTRA: from the term *man* (mind) and *tra* (transport or vehicle). It is a powerful sound or vibration that can be used to enter deep states of meditation.

Manipura: is the solar plexus, the 3rd chakra, located in the diaphragm. It is associated with the fire element and the need for power and significance.

Muladhara: is the root chakra, the 1st chakra, located at the base of the spine. It is associated with security and grounding.

Nasyam: a treatment for nose, throat, sinuses and head where medicine is given through the nostrils.

Ojas: can be understood as the terminal product of dhatus that are formed as a result of progressive metabolic processes. It is taken up in Ayurveda as the premium quality end product of normal metabolism of food and nutrients consumed in a wholesome manner. It is an Ayurvedic index of perfect health. The quantity of ojas will determine the state of health.

Pancha: 5.

Panchakarma: the classical Ayurvedic cleansing process for body and mind. *Pancha* means 5 and *karma* means actions/procedures. Panchakarma includes 5 procedures to eliminate the vitiated doshas and toxins from body and mind.

Pitta: the bioenergy controlled by fire with a small amount of water.

Prakriti: the essential nature of a human being.

Prana: the life force that enters the body at birth, travels through all the parts of the body until it leaves at the moment of death. It is the subtle form of *vata*.

Pranayama: breathing technics.

Rajas: the mind quality which characterises change, activity, the transformation from darkness to light and from light to darkness. It creates a lot of emotion, turbulence, ambition and a feeling of domination.

Rasayana: rejuvenation therapy that regenerates the mind and body and prevents or reverses the ageing process.

Rishi: a wise man, an enlightened being. A messenger, who came to earth to contribute to the evolution of consciousness.

Sahasrara: is the crown chakra, the 7th chakra, located at the top of the head. It is associated with our need for higher states of consciousness and transcendence.

Samana: the aspect of *vata* that manages the digestive system.

Samskara: experience of the past anchored in the subconscious, creating habits of the mind.

Sattva: the mind quality which characterises the light, the wisdom of knowledge, intelligence, harmony, purity and clarity.

Srotas: subtle channels that are present throughout the body, comparable to the meridians of Chinese medicine. It is through these channels that nutrients and all kind of information are transported in and out of our physiologies.

Svadhistana: the sacral chakra, the 2nd chakra, located about 8 cm below the navel at the centre of the lower belly. It is associated with the water element and sensuality and creativity.

Tamas: the mind quality which characterises darkness, delusion, inertia, laziness, disease, violence, anxiety and chaos.

Tejas: the fire of the spirit, which brings energy, vitality or charisma. The subtle form of *pitta*.

Vasti: medical enema.

Vata: the bioenergy controlled by air, including also the space/ether element.

Veda: all the writings and knowledge of ancient India.

Vikriti: disease, deviation of nature.

Vishuddhi: the throat chakra, located in the centre of the neck. It is associated with the space element and the need to grow.

List of Illnesses

Abscess (cutaneous): collection of pus under the epidermis.

Abscess (dental): started frequently by an untreated pulpitis evolving and swelling above the alveolar bone and a collection of pus in the adjacent soft tissue.

Acidity (gastric): uncomfortable feeling caused by poor digestion of foods.

Acne: affliction of the hair follicles appearing mostly at puberty, characterised by black points, pustules, violet scars, or all 3 at the same time.

Aerophagia: abnormal swallowing of air outside meals. It is followed by belching.

Aggressiveness: temporary or permanent character problem, bringing on violence and hostility towards another person.

Agitation: behavioural anomaly characterised by exaggerated and disordered motor activity.

Allergy: hypersensitivity acquired by the organism due to a foreign substance that translates into an immediate but varied reaction (eczema, hives, hay fever, asthma).

Alopecia: hair or body hair loss, rapid or progressive, localised or generalised.

Amenorrhoea: insufficient or lack of menstruation, irrespective of the cause.

Angina: inflammation of the throat affecting the tonsils and often the pillars of the palate.

Anorexia: loss of appetite, irrespective of the cause.

Anosmia: loss of smell.

Antipyretic: used to prevent or fight a fever.

Anxiety: discomfort due to an imprecise fear of imminent danger and various neuro-vegetative problems (epigastric problems, respiratory oppression, sudation, etc.).

Apathy: inability to act due to physical fatigue.

Aphonia: loss of voice due to an affliction of the vocal cords (such as laryngitis) or from recurring nerve paralysis.

Arrhythmia: irregular heartbeat.

Arthritis: inflammation of the synovial membrane of a joint.

Arthrosis: destruction of joint cartilage via mechanical use. It is localised and does not alter the general state of the subject.

Asthenia: reduction of power and strength, of nervous, psychic, physical or sexual origins.

Asthma (allergic and nervous): a disease characterised by recurrent attacks of breathlessness and wheezing, which vary in severity and frequency from person to person.

Atherosclerosis: the build-up of a waxy plaque on the inside of blood vessels. It is a progressive process, responsible for most heart diseases.

Bronchitis (acute): acute inflammation of the tracheobronchial tree, more frequent in winter. It can appear after a cold or a viral infection of the nasopharynx, the throat or the bronchi.

Bronchitis (asthmatic): association of bronchitis with a chronic cough and continuous dyspnoea asthma.

Bronchitis (chronic): permanent or intermittent cough lasting for a minimum of 3 months per year over a period of at least 2 years.

Burn: tissue lesion linked to a thermal, chemical or electrical source; first degree (simple yet painful erythema); second degree (blisters containing fibrinous exudate, sensitive to the touch); third degree (carbonisation of teguments and surrounding areas, hypoesthesia or anaesthesia of the burnt zone).

Candidiasis (cutaneous): affliction of the *Candida* group (normally *Candida albicans*) localised on the skin.

Candidiasis (vaginal): affliction of the *Candida* group (normally *Candida albicans*) affecting the vaginal mucosa.

Cellulite: inflammation of the subcutaneous cell tissue. This term is commonly used to designate, often in women, the excessive development of fatty subcutaneous tissue leading to ungainly and painful dimpling of the thighs and sides (orange peel appearance).

Cholesterol: fatty substance that is normally found in bile and blood. It comes from food but the liver also synthesises it. It is indispensable for life, as it allows for the development of sexual hormones, adrenaline and bile acid.

CIRRHOSIS: illness caused by the degeneration of the liver cells as fibrosis sets in. The main cause is alcoholism.

COLD: general inflammation of the respiratory tract mucosa (nose, throat, bronchi).

COLITIS: inflammatory state of the colon lining. The origin is mechanic, bacterial or amoebic. It is followed by alternating diarrhoea and constipation.

CONJUNCTIVITIS: inflammation of the conjunctiva (transparent membrane that covers the eye and the internal part of the eyelids). The origins are microbial, viral or allergic.

CONSTIPATION: infrequent or difficult emission of stool.

COUGH (SPASMODIC): coughing at very close intervals, provoking spasms of the diaphragm, making it difficult to breathe deeply.

CROHN'S DISEASE: affliction of the digestive tube, normally found in the ileum. The lesions are followed/alternate with healthy zones.

CYSTITIS: inflammation and/or infection of the bladder provoking the frequent and painful need to urinate.

DANDRUFF: fine flakes of skin that fall off the scalp.

DYSMENORRHOEA: painful problems with the flow of menstrual periods.

DYSPEPSIA: difficult and painful digestion.

ECZEMA: cutaneous affliction characterised by very itchy red plaques, covered with small vesicles that form crusts and scales. Frequently it is due to an external cause linked to an allergic manifestation following contact with a substance.

EMMENAGOGUE: this favours or regularises period flow.

ENTEROCOLITIS: inflammation of the small intestinal wall and the colon.

ENURESIS: involuntary urination, especially at night, in children over 4, where their urinary tract structure does not show anomalies.

FEVER BLISTER (LABIAL HERPES): recurring viral infection characterised by the appearance on the labial mucosa of isolated or multiple groups of small vesicles with clear contents, resting on a slightly raised inflammatory base.

HOT FLASHES: due to hormone change during menopause. Typically experienced as a feeling of intense heat with sweating and rapid heartbeat, and may typically last from 2 to 30 minutes.

DELIVERY (EASING OF): easing the expulsion of the foetus and placenta from the genital tract.

Depression: pathological psychic state associating a painful modification of mood and a slowing of intellectual and motor activity.

Diabetes: illness where sugar increases in the blood and urine. Its origins are a defect in the secretion or use of insulin (hormone) secreted in the pancreas.

Diarrhoea (infectious): increase in the volume, fluidity and frequency of stool compared to normal. Its origins are of an infectious digestive character.

Distention: bloating of the stomach caused by intestinal gas.

Epicondylitis: inflammation of the articulating part of the protruding bone in the elbow.

Epistaxis: nose bleed, nasal haemorrhage.

Fatigue (nervous): nervous state in which the subject reacts to a situation with excessive verbal or physical violence compared to normal.

Fatigue (physical): state in which the subject has difficulty acting. This fatigue intervenes after a prolonged or excessive effort.

Fibroid (uterine): benign fibrous tumour that develops in the uterus.

Flatulence: presence of gastric and intestinal gas provoking a swelling of the stomach or intestine.

Flu: infectious and contagious illness linked to myxovirus influenza A, B and C, evolving in the form of major pandemics combined with small seasonal and localised epidemics with variable severity.

Gastralgia: pain in the stomach.

Gastritis: affliction characterised by inflammation of the stomach's mucosa.

Gingivitis: affliction characterised by inflammation of the gums.

Gout: illness caused by an overabundance of uric acid in the body. It is characterised by painful joints, normally starting with the large toe.

Hay fever: an allergic condition affecting the mucous membranes of the upper respiratory tract and the eyes, most often characterised by nasal discharge, sneezing and itchy, watery eyes, and usually caused by an abnormal sensitivity to airborne pollen.

Heavy legs: impression of lack of lightness and bloating of the legs due to poor circulation.

Hepatic colic: pain in the right hypochondria or the epigastrium, which moves to the right shoulder, associated with nausea. The cause is often biliary lithiasis.

Haematoma: collection of blood under the skin causing large stains, purplish with irregular contours. They normally disappear after several days. Also known as bruises.

Haemorrhage: effusion of blood outside the veins. It is always a pathological state, except for menstruation.

Haemorrhoids: enlarged veins in the anus or lower rectum. They often go unnoticed and usually clear up after a few days, but can cause long-lasting discomfort and bleeding and be excruciatingly painful.

Hepatitis (viral): hepatic attack of viral origins with pathogen agents have a predominant hepatotropism (A, IH, B or SH virus).

Herpes (genital): genital herpes is a sexually transmitted disease caused by a herpes virus. The disease is characterised by the formation of fluid-filled, painful blisters in the genital area.

Herpes (labial): also called fever blister or cold sore, a type of infection occurring on the lip caused by herpes simplex virus (HSV). An outbreak typically causes small blisters or sores on or around the mouth.

Hiccups: a spasmodic and uncontrolled contraction of the diaphragm, translating into a brutal thoracoabdominal spasm followed by a characteristic sound given off by the glottis.

Hives: pinkish or red swelling of the skin, in layers, and accompanied by itching.

Hyperkinesia: normally referred to in children who have an uncontrollable need to move constantly; they lack concentration as long as they are subjected to external stimuli.

Hypertension: an increase in blood pressure above the normal level.

Hyperthyroidism: hypersecreting of thyroidal hormones.

Hypotension: abnormal lowering of blood pressure.

Hypothyroidism: failure to secrete thyroidal hormones.

Immunity: humoral and cellular factors that protect the body from toxic or infectious attacks.

Impetigo: microbial cutaneous infection (staphylococcus or streptococcus) characterised by crusty lesions on the face and hands, which can become generalised.

Indigestion: digestive/gastric problems not related to a lesion in the stomach.

Insomnia: difficulty falling asleep.

Laryngitis: acute or chronic inflammation of the lining of the laryngeal and vocal cords translating into a modification of the voice or complete aphonia.

LAXITY OF JOINTS: serious relaxation of the pressure and resistance of ligaments.

MALE DYSFUNCTION: inability for males to have an erection or maintain an erection allowing for normal sex. The cause can be motor-based or psychological.

MOTION SICKNESS: all problems observed (nausea, vertigo, tinnitus) in passengers of a moving vehicle.

MASTITIS: inflammation of breast tissue.

MENOPAUSE: cessation of ovarian activities and the total disappearance of menstruation in women.

MENORRHAGIA: abnormally abundant periods that prolong beyond their normal length.

METRITIS: inflammation of the uterus.

MIGRAINE: intense headache, characterised by strong pain in the head.

MULTIPLE SCLEROSIS: affliction of the nervous system and the spinal cord, slowly progressive, characterised by a localised demyelination of the white matter. Very polymorphic neurological signs evolve in spurt and remission phases.

MYALGIA: pain in the nerve paths.

MYCOSIS (CUTANEOUS): fungal infection of the epidermis, even the dermis.

MYCOSIS (NAIL): nail fungal infection.

NEPHRITIC COLIC: painful and violent attack in the lumbar region, generally radiating out to the thigh and lower stomach. The most frequent cause is ureteral lithiasis (stones in the passage between the kidney and bladder).

NEPHRITIS: kidney inflammation.

NEURITIS: nerve lesion.

OBESITY: excess body fat, overweight.

OEDEMA: (also edema, dropsy and hydropsy) an abnormal accumulation of fluid in the interstitium, located beneath the skin and in the cavities of the body. Clinically, oedema manifests as swelling. The amount of interstitial fluid is determined by the balance of fluid homeostasis, and the increased secretion of fluid into the interstitium or the impaired removal of the fluid can cause oedema.

OESTROGEN: hormones that stimulate the growth of female genital organs, mammary glands and vaginal secretions during the cycle. A lack of oestrogen can lead to amenorrhoea, a lack of fertility, and menopausal problems.

OESTROGEN-LIKE: substance that resembles oestrogen in its molecular structure.

OLIGURIA: lowering of the quantity of urine released over a 24-hour period.

Photosensitivity: reaction of the skin to light; the cutaneous parts exposed present redness when exposed to the sun's rays.

Polyarthritis (rheumatoid): particularly seen in women, affecting the synovial membranes of joints, leading to their destruction.

Polyneuritis: affliction affecting several peripheral nerves.

Post-partum: after birth.

Premenstrual syndrome (PMS): all of the manifestations occurring with certain women several days before their periods: painful sensitivity of the uterus and ovaries, abdominal bloating, pressure in the breasts, irritability, depression, insomnia, migraines and hot flashes.

Progesterone: hormone secreted during the post-ovulatory period of the cycle and during pregnancy. It is used in the treatment of menorrhagia and menopausal problems, as well in certain cases of sterility and to prevent miscarriages.

Prostatitis: acute or chronic inflammation of the prostate.

Pruritus: strong and violent itching.

Psoriasis: benign erythmatosquamosus dermatosis localised on the elbows, knees, lower back and scalp.

Pulpitis: inflammation of the tooth's soft tissue, pulp.

Pyelonephritis: association of interstitial microbial nephritis, an inflammation of the pelvis and a urinary infection.

Pyorrhoea: alveolar-dental inflammation with the formation of pus, provoking the loosening of the teeth and often leading to them falling out.

Raynaud's disease: also called Raynaud's phenomenon, it is a condition that affects the blood vessels. There will be periods where the body does not send blood to the hands and feet. This happens especially when the climate is cold or in case of stress. During an attack, fingers and toes may feel very cold or numb.

Rheumatism: Chronic inflammation and pain of joints and connective tissue. The term covers many different conditions such as arthritis, arthrosis and osteoarthritis.

Rosacea: red colouration of the face due to the dilatation of capillary veins.

Sciatica: very painful affliction of the sciatic nerve.

Seborrhoea: hypersecreting of sebum.

Sinusitis: acute or chronic inflammation of a facial sinus. There can also be a subjacent effect on the periosteum.

Sore: superficial ulceration of the mucosa that is painful (buccal or genital).

Shingles: infectious disease due to a chicken-pox/shingles virus, which manifests itself as eruptions of the vesicles along a nerve's path. The after effects are painful.

Shock: violent and brutal emotion bringing on an injury to the person's morale.

Spasmophilia: neuromuscular over-excitement manifesting in cramps, tingling, agitation attacks and discomfort.

Stomatitis: inflammation of the mouth mucosa.

Stress: also refers to the tension or attack against the organism, or the non-specific response or reaction of the organism to this assault.

Teething pain: pain linked to the growth of a new tooth bringing on the perforation of the gums and a reorganisation of the adjacent tissues (soft and hard tissue, nerves, veins, etc.).

Tennis elbow: see epicondylitis.

Thrombosis: the inflammation of a vein that can lead to the formation of a clot.

Thrush: illness in the buccal mucosa in particular, brought on by a mushroom. Whitish plaques appear, as well as an acidic reaction of the saliva.

Urethritis: affliction of the urethra, due to the inflammation of its mucosa.

Vascular fragility: lack of resistance of the veins.

Vaginal infection: affliction due to the inflammation of the vagina.

Varicose vein: permanent dilation of a vein that has lost its natural elasticity and pathological alteration of its walls.

Vulvitis: inflammation of the vulva.

Wound: an injury, usually involving division of tissue or rupture of the integument or mucous membrane, due to external violence or some mechanical agency rather than disease.

Therapeutic Index

Properties	Hydrosols
Ajna (activating the 6th chakra)	Cistus (*Cistus ladaniferus*) Eucalyptus (*Eucalyptus globulus*) Everlasting (*Helichrysum italicum*) Hyssop (*Hyssopus off. officinalis*) Ravintsara (*Cinnamomum camphora*) Sage (*Salvia officinalis*) Sandalwood (*Santalum album*)
Anahata (activating the 4th chakra)	Champak (*Michelia alba*) Kewra (*Pandanus odoratus*) Lemon verbena (*Lippia citriodora*) Marjoram (*Origanum majorana*) Myrtle (*Myrtus communis*) Palmarosa (*Cymbopogon martinii*) Rose (*Rosa damascena*) Spikenard (*Nardostachys jatamansi*) Thyme linalool (*Thymus vulgaris linaloliferum*)

Analgesic	Angelica root (*Angelica archangelica*)
	Atlas cedar (*Cedrus atlanticum*)
	Basil (*Ocimum basilicum*)
	Bay laurel (*Laurus nobilis*)
	Bergamot (*Citrus bergamia*)
	Blue camomile (*Camomilla matricaria*)
	Champaca (*Michelia alba*)
	Cinnamon (*Cinnamomum verum*)
	Clary sage (*Salvia sclarea*)
	Coriander (*Coriandrum sativum*)
	Frankincense (*Boswellia carterii*)
	Geranium (*Pelargonium asperum*)
	Jasmine (*Jasminum officinalis*)
	Kewra (*Pandanus odoratissimus*)
	Lavender (*Lavandula vera*)
	Lemon verbena (*Lippia citriodora*)
	Marjoram (*Origanum majorana*)
	Orange blossom (*Citrus aurantium*)
	Palmarosa (*Cymbopogon martinii*)
	Peppermint (*Mentha piperita*)
	Ravintsara (*Cinnamomum camphora*)
	Roman camomile (*Chamaemelum nobile*)
	Rose (*Rosa damascena*)
	Sage (*Salvia officinalis*)
	Sandalwood (*Santalum album*)
	Scots pine (*Pinus sylvestris*)
	Shiso (*Perilla frutescens*)
	Spikenard (*Nardostachys jatamansi*)
	St John's wort (*Hypericum perforatum*)
	Thyme thymol (*Thymus vulgaris thymoliferum*)
	Yarrow (*Achillea millefolium*)
	Ylang ylang (*Cananga odorata*)
Anti-premature contractions	Kewra (*Pandanus odoratus*)

Antiacid	Coriander (*Coriandrum sativum*)
	Kewra (*Pandanus odoratissimus*)
	Lavender (*Lavandula vera*)
	Peppermint (*Mentha piperita*)
	Rose (*Rosa damascena*)
Anti-allergic	Blue camomile (*Camomilla matricaria*)
	Myrtle (*Myrtus communis*)
	Roman camomile (*Chamaemelum nobile*)
	Shiso (*Perilla frutescens*)
	St John's wort (*Hypericum perforatum*)
	Yarrow (*Achillea millefolium*)
Anti-asthmatic	Angelica root (*Angelica archangelica*)
	Atlas cedar (*Cedrus atlanticum*)
	Basil (*Ocimum basilicum*)
	Blue camomile (*Camomilla matricaria*)
	Myrtle (*Myrtus communis*)
	Frankincense (*Boswellia carterii*)
	Hyssop (*Hyssopus officinalis*)
	Sage (*Salvia officinalis*)
	Scots pine (*Pinus sylvestris*)
	Shiso (*Perilla frutescens*)

Antibacterial	Bay laurel (*Laurus nobilis*)
	Bergamot (*Citrus bergamia*)
	Cinnamon (*Cinnamomum verum*)
	Cistus (*Cistus ladaniferus*)
	Coriander (*Coriandrum sativum*)
	Geranium (*Pelargonium asperum*)
	Marjoram (*Origanum majorana*)
	Myrtle (*Myrtus communis*)
	Palmarosa (*Cymbopogon martinii*)
	Rose (*Rosa damascena*)
	Sage (*Salvia officinalis*)
	Savory (*Satureja montana*)
	Shiso (*Perilla frutescens*)
	Tea tree (*Melaleuca alternifolia*)
	Thyme linalool (*Thymus vulgaris linaloliferum*)
	Thyme thymol (*Thymus vulgaris thymoliferum*)
Anti-cough	Cistus (*Cistus ladaniferus*)
	Cypress (*Cupressus sempervirens*)
	Myrtle (*Myrtus communis*)
	Ravintsara (*Cinnamomum camphora*)
	Rose (*Rosa damascena*)
	Sage (*Salvia officinalis*)
	Scots pine (*Pinus sylvestris*)

Anti-depressant	Angelica root (*Angelica archangelica*)
	Bergamot (*Citrus bergamia*)
	Champaca (*Michelia alba*)
	Cinnamon (*Cinnamomum verum*)
	Clary sage (*Salvia sclarea*)
	Geranium (*Pelargonium asperum*)
	Jasmine (*Jasminum officinalis*)
	Kewra (*Pandanus odoratissimus*)
	Lavender (*Lavandula vera*)
	Lemon verbena (*Lippia citriodora*)
	Orange blossom (*Citrus aurantium*)
	Ravintsara (*Cinnamomum camphora*)
	Roman camomile (*Chamaemelum nobile*)
	Rose (*Rosa damascena*)
	Sandalwood (*Santalum album*)
	St John's wort (*Hypericum perforatum*)
	Ylang ylang (*Cananga odorata*)
Anti-diabetic	Angelica root (*Angelica archangelica*)
	Atlas cedar (*Cedrus atlanticum*)
	Carrot (*Daucus carota*)
	Coriander (*Coriandrum sativum*)
	Eucalyptus (*Eucalyptus globulus*)
	Everlasting (*Helichrysum italicum*)
	Frankincense (*Boswellia carterii*)
	Geranium (*Pelargonium asperum*)
	Kewra (*Pandanus odoratissimus*)
	Scots pine (*Pinus sylvestris*)
	Shiso (*Perilla frutescens*)
Anti-epileptic	Kewra (*Pandanus odoratus*)
	Shiso (*Perilla frutescens*)
Anti-haematoma	Everlasting (*Helichrysum italicum*)
Anti-haemorrhagic	Cistus (*Cistus ladaniferus*)
	Geranium (*Pelargonium asperum*)
	Yarrow (*Achillea millefolium*)

Anti-inflammatory	Angelica root (*Angelica archangelica*)
	Bay laurel (*Laurus nobilis*)
	Bergamot (*Citrus bergamia*)
	Blue camomile (*Camomilla matricaria*)
	Carrot (*Daucus carota*)
	Champaca (*Michelia alba*)
	Cinnamon (*Cinnamomum verum*)
	Cistus (*Cistus ladaniferus*)
	Clary sage (*Salvia sclarea*)
	Coriander (*Coriandrum sativum*)
	Everlasting (*Helichrysum italicum*)
	Frankincense (*Boswellia carterii*)
	Geranium (*Pelargonium asperum*)
	Juniper (*Juniperus communis*)
	Kewra (*Pandanus odoratus*)
	Lavender (*Lavandula vera*)
	Ledum (*Rhododendron groenlandicum*)
	Marjoram (*Origanum majorana*)
	Myrtle (*Myrtus communis*)
	Palmarosa (*Cymbopogon martinii*)
	Peppermint (*Mentha piperita*)
	Ravintsara (*Cinnamomum camphora*)
	Roman camomile (*Chamaemelum nobilis*)
	Rose (*Rosa damascena*)
	Sage (*Salvia officinalis*)
	Sandalwood (*Santalum album*)
	Scots pine (*Pinus sylvestris*)
	Shiso (*Perilla frutescens*)
	Spikenard (*Nardostachys jatamansi*)
	St John's wort (*Hypericum perforatum*)
	Verbena (*Lippia citriodora*)
	Yarrow (*Achillea millefolium*)
	Ylang ylang (*Cananga odorata*)
Anti-neuralgia	Yarrow (*Achillea millefolium*)

Antioxidant	Eucalyptus (*Eucalyptus globulus*)
	Kewra (*Pandanus odoratus*)
	Rose (*Rosa damascena*)
	Rosemary verbenon (*Rosmarinus verbenoniferum*)
	Sage (*Salvia officinalis*)
	Shiso (*Perilla frutescens*)
Anti-parasitic	Atlas cedar (*Cedrus atlanticum*)
	Coriander (*Coriandrum sativum*)
	Geranium (*Pelargonium asperum*)
	Lavender (*Lavandula vera*)
	Palmarosa (*Cymbopogon martinii*)
	Roman camomile (*Chamaemelum nobile*)
	Rosemary verbenon (*Rosmarinus verbenoniferum*)
	Sage (*Salvia officinalis*)
	Savory (*Satureja montana*)
	Thyme linalool (*Thymus vulgaris linaloliferum*)
	Thyme thymol (*Thymus vulgaris thymoliferum*)
Antiperspirant	Sage (*Salvia officinalis*)
Antiseptic	Bay laurel (*Laurus nobilis*)
	Cinnamon (*Cinnamomum verum*)
	Cistus (*Cistus ladaniferus*)
	Eucalyptus (*Eucalyptus globulus*)
	Frankincense (*Boswellia carterii*)
	Geranium (*Pelargonium asperum*)
	Jasmine (*Jasminum officinalis*)
	Juniper (*Juniperus communis*)
	Kewra (*Pandanus odoratus*)
	Myrtle (*Myrtus communis*)
	Palmarosa (*Cymbopogon martinii*)
	Ravintsara (*Cinnamomum camphora*)
	Rose (*Rosa damascena*)
	Sandalwood (*Santalum album*)
	Scots pine (*Pinus sylvestris*)
	Thyme linalool (*Thymus vulgaris linaloliferum*)
	Ylang ylang (*Cananga odorata*)

Antispasmodic	Angelica root (*Angelica archangelica*)
	Basil (*Ocimum basilicum*)
	Bay laurel (*Laurus nobilis*)
	Bergamot (*Citrus bergamia*)
	Champaca (*Michelia champaca*)
	Clary sage (*Salvia sclarea*)
	Coriander (*Coriandrum sativum*)
	Frankincense (*Boswellia carterii*)
	Geranium (*Pelargonium asperum*)
	Kewra (*Pandanus odoratissimus*)
	Lavender (*Lavandula vera*)
	Lemon verbena (*Lippia citriodora*)
	Orange blossom (*Citrus aurantium*)
	Palmarosa (*Cymbopogon martinii*)
	Ravintsara (*Cinnamomum camphora*)
	Roman camomile (*Chamaemelum nobile*)
	Rose (*Rosa damascena*)
	Scots pine (*Pinus sylvestris*)
	Spikenard (*Nardostachys jatamansi*)
	St John's wort (*Hypericum perforatum*)
	Yarrow (*Achillea millefolium*)
	Ylang ylang (*Cananga odorata*)
Anti-stress	Bergamot (*Citrus bergamia*)
	Champaca (*Michelia alba*)
	Clary sage (*Salvia sclarea*)
	Geranium (*Pelargonium asperum*)
	Kewra (*Pandanus odoratissimus*)
	Lavender (*Lavandula vera*)
	Lemon verbena (*Lippia citriodora*)
	Marjoram (*Origanum majorana*)
	Orange blossom (*Citrus aurantium*)
	Palmarosa (*Cymbopogon martinii*)
	Ravintsara (*Cinnamomum camphora*)
	Rose (*Rosa damascena*)
	Spikenard (*Nardostachys jatamansi*)
	St John's wort (*Hypericum perforatum*)
	Vetiver (*Vetiveria zizanoides*)
	Ylang ylang (*Cananga odorata*)

Anxiolytic	Bergamot (*Citrus bergamia*)
	Clary sage (*Salvia sclarea*)
	Jasmine (*Jasminum officinalis*)
	Marjoram (*Origanum majorana*)
	Orange blossom (*Citrus aurantium*)
	Palmarosa (*Cymbopogon martinii*)
	Ravintsara (*Cinnamomum camphora*)
	Rose (*Rosa damascena*)
	Spikenard (*Nardostachys jatamansi*)
	St John's wort (*Hypericum perforatum*)
	Lemon verbena (*Lippia citriodora*)
	Vetiver (*Vetiveria zizanoides*)
	Ylang ylang (*Cananga odorata*)
Aphrodisiac	Bergamot (*Citrus bergamia*)
	Champaca (*Michelia alba*)
	Cinnamon (*Cinnamomum verum*)
	Frankincense (*Boswellia carterii*)
	Jasmine (*Jasminum officinalis*)
	Kewra (*Pandanus odoratus*)
	Rose (*Rosa damascena*)
	Sandalwood (*Santalum album*)
	Ylang ylang (*Cananga odorata*)
Appetite stimulant	Bergamot (*Citrus bergamia*)
Astringent	Atlas cedar (*Cedrus atlanticum*)
	Bergamot (*Citrus bergamia*)
	Cistus (*Cistus ladaniferus*)
	Cypress (*Cupressus sempervirens*)
	Jasmine (*Jasminum officinalis*)
	Lavender (*Lavandula vera*)
	Myrtle (*Myrtus communis*)
	Palmarosa (*Cymbopogon martinii*)
	Peppermint (*Mentha piperita*)
	Rose (*Rosa damascena*)
	Rosemary verbenon (*Rosmarinus off. verbenoniferum*)
	Sage (*Salvia officinalis*)
	Sandalwood (*Santalum album*)
	Scots pine (*Pinus sylvestris*)

Blood purifier	Everlasting (*Helichrysum italicum*)
Blood thinner	Angelica root (*Angelica archangelica*)
	Everlasting (*Helichrysum italicum*)
	Lemon verbena (*Lippia citriodora*)
Calming	Blue camomile (*Camomilla matricaria*)
	Jasmine (*Jasminum officinalis*)
	Lemon verbena (*Lippia citriodora*)
	Marjoram (*Origanum majorana*)
	Orange blossom (*Citrus aurantium*)
	Palmarosa (*Cymbopogon martinii*)
	Ravintsara (*Cinnamomum camphora*)
	Roman camomile (*Chamaemelum nobile*)
	Rose (*Rosa damascena*)
	Sandalwood (*Santalum album*)
	Spikenard (*Nardostachys jatamansi*)
	St John's wort (*Hypericum perforatum*)
	Vetiver (*Vetiveria zizanoides*)
	Ylang ylang (*Cananga odorata*)
Cardiotonic	Atlas cedar (*Cedrus atlanticum*)
	Champaca (*Michelia alba*)
	Cinnamon (*Cinnamomum verum*)
	Coriander (*Coriandrum sativum*)
	Frankincense (*Boswellia carterii*)
	Geranium (*Pelargonium asperum*)
	Kewra (*Pandanus odoratus*)
	Palmarosa (*Cymbopogon martinii*)
	Rose (*Rosa damascena*)
	Sandalwood (*Santalum album*)
	Spikenard (*Nardostachys jatamansi*)
	Vetiver (*Vetiveria zizanoides*)
	Ylang ylang (*Cananga odorata*)

Cardiovascular regenerator	Carrot (*Daucus carota*)
	Kewra (*Pandanus odoratus*)
	Lavender (*Lavandula vera*)
	Lemon verbena (*Lippia citriodora*)
	Orange blossom (*Citrus aurantium*)
	Palmarosa (*Cymbopogon martinii*)
	Rose (*Rosa damascena*)
	Spikenard (*Nardostachys jatamansi*)
	Ylang ylang (*Cananga odorata*)
Carminative	Angelica root (*Angelica archangelica*)
	Bay laurel (*Laurus nobilis*)
	Bergamot (*Citrus bergamia*)
	Frankincense (*Boswellia carterii*)
	Rosemary verbenon (*Rosmarinus off. verbenoniferum*)
	Spikenard (*Nardostachys jatamansi*)
Circulatory and lymphatic stimulant	Cypress (*Cupressus sempervirens*)
	Everlasting (*Helichrysum italicum*)
	Juniper (*Juniperus communis*)
	Rosemary verbenon (*Rosmarinus off. verbenoniferum*)
	Sage (*Salvia officinalis*)
	Sandalwood (*Santalum album*)
	Scots pine (*Pinus sylvestris*)
	Tea tree (*Melaleuca alternifolia*)
	Vetiver (*Vetiveria zizanoides*)
	Yarrow (*Achillea millefolium*)
Cutaneous firming	Cistus (*Cistus ladaniferus*)
	Rose (*Rosa damascena*)
	Rosemary verbenon (*Rosmarinus off. verbenoniferum*)
	Spikenard (*Nardostachys jatamansi*)
	Vetiver (*Vetiveria zizanoides*)
	Ylang ylang (*Cananga odorata*)

Cutaneous regeneration	Atlas cedar (*Cedrus atlanticum*)
	Carrot (*Daucus carota*)
	Champaca (*Michelia alba*)
	Frankincense (*Boswellia carterii*)
	Kewra (*Pandanus odoratus*)
	Orange blossom (*Citrus aurantium*)
	Rose (*Rosa damascena*)
	Sage (*Salvia officinalis*)
	Spikenard (*Nardostachys jatamansi*)
	Vetiver (*Vetiveria zizanoides*)
	Ylang ylang (*Cananga odorata*)
Depurative	Angelica root (*Angelica archangelica*)
	Atlas cedar (*Cedrus atlanticum*)
	Carrot (*Daucus carota*)
	Cypress (*Cupressus sempervirens*)
	Eucalyptus (*Eucalyptus globulus*)
	Geranium (*Pelargonium asperum*)
	Juniper (*Juniperus communis*)
	Kewra (*Pandanus odoratus*)
	Ledum (*Rhododendron groenlandicum*)
	Rose (*Rosa damascena*)
	Rosemary verbenon (*Rosmarinus off. verbenoniferum*)
	Sage (*Salvia officinalis*)
	Savory (*Satureja montana*)
	Scots pine (*Pinus sylvestris*)
	Shiso (*Perilla frutescens*)

Digestive	Angelica root (*Angelica archangelica*)
	Basil (*Ocimum basilicum*)
	Bay laurel (*Laurus nobilis*)
	Bergamot (*Citrus bergamia*)
	Cinnamon (*Cinnamomum verum*)
	Lavender (*Lavandula vera*)
	Marjoram (*Origanum majorana*)
	Rose (*Rosa damascena*)
	Rosemary verbenon (*Rosmarinus off. verbenoniferum*)
	Sage (*Salvia officinalis*)
	Sandalwood (*Santalum album*)
	Scots pine (*Pinus sylvestris*)
	Shiso (*Perilla frutescens*)
	Spikenard (*Nardostachys jatamansi*)
	Vetiver (*Vetiveria zizanoides*)
	Yarrow (*Achillea millefolium*)
Diuretic	Cinnamon (*Cinnamomum verum*)
	Frankincense (*Boswellia carterii*)
	Jasmine (*Jasminum officinalis*)
	Juniper (*Juniperus communis*)
	Rosemary verbenon (*Rosmarinus off. verbenoniferum*)
	Sage (*Salvia officinalis*)
	Sandalwood (*Santalum album*)
	Scots pine (*Pinus sylvestris*)
	Spikenard (*Nardostachys jatamansi*)
Emmenagogue	Bay laurel (*Laurus nobilis*)
	Clary sage (*Salvia sclarea*)
	Jasmine (*Jasminum officinalis*)
	Palmarosa (*Cymbopogon martinii*)
	Sage (*Salvia officinalis*)
	Spikenard (*Nardostachys jatamansi*)
	Vetiver (*Vetiveria zizanoides*)

Expectorant	Angelica root (*Angelica archangelica*)
	Eucalyptus (*Eucalyptus globulus*)
	Frankincense (*Boswellia carterii*)
	Jasmine (*Jasminum officinalis*)
	Myrtle (*Myrtus communis*)
	Ravintsara (*Cinnamomum camphora*)
	Rose (*Rosa damascena*)
	Rosemary verbenon (*Rosmarinus off. verbenoniferum*)
	Sage (*Salvia officinalis*)
	Scots pine (*Pinus sylvestris*)
	Yarrow (*Achillea millefolium*)
Eye decongestant	Myrtle (*Myrtus communis*)
	Rose (*Rosa damascena*)
Fungicidal	Bay laurel (*Laurus nobilis*)
	Bergamot (*Citrus bergamia*)
	Cinnamon (*Cinnamomum verum*)
	Coriander (*Coriandrum sativum*)
	Geranium (*Pelargonium asperum*)
	Marjoram (*Origanum majorana*)
	Myrtle (*Myrtus communis*)
	Palmarosa (*Cymbopogon martinii*)
	Rose (*Rosa damascena*)
	Sage (*Salvia officinalis*)
	Savory (*Satureja montana*)
	Scots pine (*Pinus sylvestris*)
	Tea tree (*Melaleuca alternifolia*)
	Thyme linalool (*Thymus vulgaris linaloliferum*)
	Thyme thymol (*Thymus vulgaris thymoliferum*)
	Ylang ylang (*Cananga odorata*)

Hepatic stimulant	Angelica root (*Angelica archangelica*)
	Bergamot (*Citrus bergamia*)
	Common juniper (*Juniperus communis*)
	Cypress (*Cupressus sempervirens*)
	Eucalyptus (*Eucalyptus globulus*)
	Geranium (*Pelargonium asperum*)
	Ledum (*Rhododendron groenlandicum*)
	Lemon verbena (*Lippia citriodora*)
	Rosemary verbenon (*Rosmarinus off. verbenoniferum*)
	Sage (*Salvia officinalis*)
	Vetiver (*Vetiveria zizanoides*)
Hormonal balancer for women	Cypress (*Cupressus sempervirens*)
	Geranium (*Pelargonium asperum*)
	Rose (*Rosa damascena*)
	Sage (*Salvia officinalis*)
	Spikenard (*Nardostachys jatamansi*)
	Vetiver (*Vetiveria zizanoides*)
	Yarrow (*Achillea millefolium*)
Hypertensor	Rosemary verbenon (*Rosmarinus off. verbenoniferum*)
	Savory (*Satureja montana*)
	Thyme thymol (*Thymus vulgaris thymoliferum*)
Hypotensor	Lavender (*Lavandula vera*)
	Marjoram (*Origanum majorana*)
	Rose (*Rosa damascena*)
	Sandalwood (*Santalum album*)
	Spikenard (*Nardostachys jatamansi*)
	Ylang ylang (*Cananga odorata*)

Immune booster	Angelica root (*Angelica archangelica*)
	Cinnamon (*Cinnamomum verum*)
	Cistus (*Cistus ladaniferus*)
	Coriander (*Coriandrum sativum*)
	Frankincense (*Boswellia carterii*)
	Kewra (*Pandanus odoratus*)
	Myrtle (*Myrtus communis*)
	Palmarosa (*Cymbopogon martinii*)
	Ravintsara (*Cinnamomum camphora*)
	Rose (*Rosa damascena*)
	Sandalwood (*Santalum album*)
	Savory (*Satureja montana*)
	Scots pine (*Pinus sylvestris*)
	Shiso (*Perilla frutescens*)
	Tea tree (*Melaleuca alternifolia*)
	Thyme linalool (*Thymus vulgaris linaloliferum*)
	Thyme thymol (*Thymus vulgaris thymoliferum*)
	Vetiver (*Vetiveria zizanoides*)
Kidney and gallbladder regenerator	Rose (*Rosa damascena*)
	Rosemary verbenon (*Rosmarinus off. verbenoniferum*)
	Sage (*Salvia officinalis*)
Kidney stimulant	Cypress (*Cupressus sempervirens*)
	Eucalyptus (*Eucalyptus globulus*)
	Juniper (*Juniperus communis*)
	Rosemary verbenon (*Rosmarinus off. verbenoniferum*)
	Sage (*Salvia officinalis*)
Litholytic	Atlas cedar (*Cedrus atlanticum*)
	Juniper (*Juniperus communis*)
	Lemon verbena (*Lippia citriodora*)
	Scots pine (*Pinus sylvestris*)
Manipura (activating the 3rd chakra)	Basil (*Ocimum basilicum*)
	Rosemary verbenon (*Rosmarinus off. verbenoniferum*)

Manipura (balancing the 3rd chakra)	Geranium (*Pelargonium asperum*)
	Ledum (*Rhododendron groenlandicum*)
	Lemon verbena (*Lippia citriodora*)
	Roman camomile (*Chamaemelum nobile*)
	St John's wort (*Hypericum perforatum*)
Metabolic stimulant	Jasmine (*Jasminum officinalis*)
	Lemon verbena (*Lippia citriodora*)
	Rosemary verbenon (*Rosmarinus off. verbenoniferum*)
	Sage (*Salvia officinalis*)
	Scots pine (*Pinus sylvestris*)
	Tea tree (*Melaleuca alternifolia*)
Mucolytic	Blue camomile (*Camomilla matricaria*)
	Eucalyptus (*Eucalyptus globulus*)
	Everlasting (*Helichrysum italicum*)
	Hyssop (*Hyssopus officinalis officinalis*)
	Juniper (*Juniperus communis*)
	Ravintsara (*Cinnamomum camphora*)
	Rose (*Rosa damascena*)
	Rosemary verbenon (*Rosmarinus off. verbenoniferum*)
	Sage (*Salvia officinalis*)
	Scots pine (*Pinus sylvestris*)
	St John's wort (*Hypericum perforatum*)
Muladhara (activating the 1st chakra)	Angelica root (*Angelica archangelica*)
	Carrot (*Daucus carota*)
	Cinnamon (*Cinnamomum verum*)
	Savory (*Satureja montana*)
	Thyme thymol (*Thymus vulgaris thymoliferum*)
	Vetiver (*Vetiveria zizanoides*)
	Vitex (*Agnus castus*)
	Yarrow (*Achillea millefolium*)

Neurotonic	Atlas cedar (*Cedrus atlanticum*)
	Blue camomile (*Camomilla matricaria*)
	Carrot (*Daucus carota*)
	Champaca (*Michelia alba*)
	Cistus (*Cistus ladaniferus*)
	Coriander (*Coriandrum sativum*)
	Jasmine (*Jasminum officinalis*)
	Kewra (*Pandanus odoratus*)
	Marjoram (*Origanum majorana*)
	Rose (*Rosa damascena*)
	Rosemary verbenon (*Rosmarinus off. verbenoniferum*)
	Sandalwood (*Santalum album*)
	Spikenard (*Nardostachys jatamansi*)
	Thyme linalool (*Thymus vulgaris linaloliferum*)
	Tea tree (*Melaleuca alternifolia*)
	Lemon verbena (*Lippia citriodora*)
	Vetiver (*Vetiveria zizanoides*)
	Vitex (*Agnus castus*)
	Ylang ylang (*Cananga odorata*)
Oestrogen-like	Clary sage (*Salvia sclarea*)
	Sage (*Salvia officinalis*)
Pancreatic stimulant	Angelica root (*Angelica archangelica*)
	Bergamot (*Citrus bergamia*)
	Common juniper (*Juniperus communis*)
	Cypress (*Cupressus sempervirens*)
	Eucalyptus (*Eucalyptus globulus*)
	Everlasting (*Helichrysum italicum*)
	Geranium (*Pelargonium asperum*)
	Lemon verbena (*Lippia citriodora*)
	Peppermint (*Mentha piperita*)
	Rosemary verbenon (*Rosmarinus off. verbenoniferum*)
	Sage (*Salvia officinalis*)
	Vetiver (*Vetiveria zizanoides*)
Progesterone-like	Rosemary verbenon (*Rosmarinus off. verbenoniferum*)
	Vitex (*Agnus castus*)

Reduces uric acid	Angelica root (*Angelica archangelica*)
	Coriander (*Coriandrum sativum*)
	Lavender (*Lavandula vera*)
	Rose (*Rosa damascena*)
	Sage (*Salvia officinalis*)
Sahasrara (activating the 7th chakra)	Atlas cedar (*Cedrus atlanticum*)
	Champaca (*Michelia alba*)
	Cypress (*Cupressus sempervirens*)
	Frankincense (*Boswellia carterii*)
	Juniper (*Juniper communis*)
	Lavender (*Lavandula vera*)
	Rose (*Rosa damascena*)
	Shiso (*Perilla frutescens*)
Sedative	Bergamot (*Citrus bergamia*)
	Lavender (*Lavandula vera*)
	Lemon verbena (*Lippia citriodora*)
	Orange blossom (*Citrus aurantium*)
	Ravintsara (*Cinnamomum camphora*)
	Spikenard (*Nardostachys jatamansi*)
	St John's wort (*Hypericum perforatum*)
	Vetiver (*Vetiveria zizanoides*)
	Ylang ylang (*Cananga odorata*)
Small basin decongestant	Clary sage (*Salvia sclarea*)
	Cypress (*Cupressus sempervirens*)
	Lemon verbena (*Lippia citriodora*)
	Rose (*Rosa damascena*)
	Sage (*Salvia officinalis*)
	Sandalwood (*Santalum album*)
	Shiso (*Perilla frutescens*)
	Vetiver (*Vetiveria zizanoides*)
	Ylang ylang (*Cananga odorata*)
Svadhistana (activating the 2nd chakra)	Bergamot (*Citrus bergamia*)
	Cistus (*Cistus ladaniferus*)
	Jasmine (*Jasminum officinalis*)
	Orange blossom (*Citrus aurantium*)
	Sandalwood (*Santalum album*)
	Ylang ylang (*Cananga odorata*)

Thyroid stimulant	Eucalyptus (*Eucalyptus globulus*)
	Lemon verbena (*Lippia citriodora*)
	Rosemary verbenon (*Rosmarinus off. verbenoniferum*)
	Scots pine (*Pinus sylvestris*)
	Tea tree (*Melaleuca alternifolia*)
Urinary decongestant	Ledum (*Rhododendron groenlandicum*)
	Lemon verbena (*Lippia citriodora*)
	Myrtle (*Myrtus communis*)
	Palmarosa (*Cymbopogon martinii*)
	Rose (*Rosa damascena*)
	Rosemary verbenon (*Rosmarinus off. verbenoniferum*)
	Sage (*Salvia officinalis*)
	Scots pine (*Pinus sylvestris*)
	Shiso (*Perilla frutescens*)
	Vetiver (*Vetiveria zizanoides*)
Uterine and ovarian regenerator	Vitex (*Agnus castus*)
Uterotonic	Cinnamon (*Cinnamomum verum*)
	Frankincense (*Boswellia carterii*)
	Jasmine (*Jasminum officinalis*)
	Lemon verbena (*Lippia citriodora*)
	Palmarosa (*Cymbopogon martinii*)
	Sage (*Salvia officinalis*)
Vasodilator	Sandalwood (*Santalum album*)
	Spikenard (*Nardostachys jatamansi*)
	Vetiver (*Vetiveria zizanoides*)
Venous decongestant	Cypress (*Cupressus sempervirens*)
	Marjoram (*Origanum majorana*)
	Rose (*Rosa damascena*)
	Rosemary verbenon (*Rosmarinus off. verbenoniferum*)
	Sage (*Salvia officinalis*)
	Sandalwood (*Santalum album*)
	Scots pine (*Pinus sylvestris*)
	Spikenard (*Nardostachys jatamansi*)
	Vetiver (*Vetiveria zizanoides*)
	Yarrow (*Achillea millefolium*)

Virucidal	Bay laurel (*Laurus nobilis*)
	Bergamot (*Citrus bergamia*)
	Coriander (*Coriandrum sativum*)
	Geranium (*Pelargonium asperum*)
	Lavender (*Lavandula vera*)
	Myrtle (*Myrtus communis*)
	Palmarosa (*Cymbopogon martinii*)
	Peppermint (*Mentha piperita*)
	Ravintsara (*Cinnamomum camphora*)
	Savory (*Satureja montana*)
	Tea tree (*Melaleuca alternifolia*)
	Thyme linalool (*Thymus vulgaris linaloliferum*)
	Thyme thymol (*Thymus vulgaris thymoliferum*)
Vishuddhi (activating the 5th chakra)	Bay laurel (*Laurus nobilis*)
	Blue camomile (*Camomilla matricaria*)
	Clary sage (*Salvia sclarea*)
	Coriander (*Coriandrum sativum*)
	Myrtle (*Myrtus communis*)
	Peppermint (*Mentha piperita*)
Wound-healing	Atlas cedar (*Cedrus atlanticum*)
	Champaca (*Michelia alba*)
	Cistus (*Cistus ladaniferus*)
	Everlasting (*Helichrysum italicum*)
	Geranium (*Pelargonium asperum*)
	Palmarosa (*Cymbopogon martinii*)
	Rose (*Rosa damascena*)
	St John's wort (*Hypericum perforatum*)
	Vetiver (*Vetiveria zizanoides*)
	Yarrow (*Achillea millefolium*)
	Ylang ylang (*Cananga odorata*)

BIBLIOGRAPHY

Catty, S. (2001) *Hydrosols: The Next Aromatherapy*. Rochester, VT: Healing Arts Press.

Emoto, M. (2005) *The Hidden Messages in Water*. New York: Atria/Simon and Schuster.

Rose, J. (1999) *375 Essential Oils and Hydrosols*. Berkeley, CA: Frog Ltd.

Price, L. and Price, S. (2004) *Understanding Hydrosols: The Specific Hydrosols for Aromatherapy. A Guide for Professionals*. Edinburgh/New York, NY: Churchill Livingstone.

Fischer-Rizzi, S. (2014) *Das Grosse Buch der Pflanzenwässer*. Aarau and Munich: AT-Verlag.